Making Individual Service Funds Work for People with Dementia Living in Care Homes

by the same author

Personalisation and Dementia
A Guide for Person-Centred Practice
Helen Sanderson and Gill Bailey
Foreword by Jeremy Hughes
ISBN 978 1 84905 379 2
eISBN 978 0 85700 734 6

A Practical Guide to Delivering Personalisation
Person-Centred Practice in Health and Social Care
Helen Sanderson and Jaimee Lewis
ISBN 978 1 84905 194 1
eISBN 978 0 85700 422 2

Creating Person-Centred Organisations
Strategies and Tools for Managing Change in Health,
Social Care and the Voluntary Sector
Stephen Stirk and Helen Sanderson
ISBN 978 1 84905 260 3
eISBN 978 0 85700 549 6

Person-Centred Teams
A Practical Guide to Delivering Personalisation
Through Effective Team-work
Helen Sanderson and Mary Beth Lepkowsky
ISBN 978 1 84905 455 3
eISBN 978 0 85700 830 5

Personalisation in Practice
Supporting Young People with Disabilities
through the Transition to Adulthood
Suzie Franklin
With Helen Sanderson
Foreword by Nicola Gitsham
ISBN 978 1 84905 443 0
eISBN 978 0 85700 816 9

Making Individual Service Funds Work for People with Dementia Living in Care Homes

How it Works in Practice

Helen Sanderson and Gill Bailey with Lisa Martin
Foreword by Dr Sam Bennett

Jessica Kingsley *Publishers*
London and Philadelphia

First published in 2014
by Jessica Kingsley Publishers
73 Collier Street
London N1 9BE, UK
and
400 Market Street, Suite 400
Philadelphia, PA 19106, USA

www.jkp.com

Library of Congress Cataloging in Publication Data
Sanderson, Helen, 1965-
  Making individual service funds work for people with dementia living in care homes : how it works in practice / Helen Sanderson and Gill Bailey with Lisa Martin.
       pages cm.
  Includes bibliographical references and index.
  ISBN 978-1-84905-545-1 (alk. paper)
  1. Medical savings accounts--Great Britain. 2. Medical care--Great Britain--Finance.
3. Dementia--Patients--Care--Great Britain. 4. Nursing homes--Patient representative services--Great Britain. I. Title.
  RA416.5.G7S26 2014
  362.160941--dc23
                                                    2014000540

British Library Cataloguing in Publication Data
A CIP catalogue record for this book is available from the British Library

ISBN 978 1 84905 545 1
eISBN 978 0 85700 975 3

Printed and bound in Great Britain by Bell and Bain Ltd, Glasgow

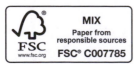

CONTENTS

Foreword

When someone's support is arranged and managed through an Individual Service Fund (ISF), they should be clear how much resource is available and be able to decide how it is used. For the provider, this should mean committing to use the majority of the money available for someone's support only on that person, rather than sinking the money into a pooled budget for a service. More fundamentally, ISFs are about changing the basis of the relationship between the provider and the person being supported, to put them firmly in the driving seat. Simple really.

Yet we have been talking about ISFs for a long time – from early pioneering work in Glasgow, through to the efforts of the individual budget pilots (my own included!) and now in the context of personalisation as mainstream policy in social care and the steady gathering of momentum for person-centred, coordinated care in health. But talking about it is one thing, doing it well and at scale is another entirely. In practice, it has often proved supremely difficult to define our terms and describe what we are talking about when we talk about ISFs, let alone to devise strategies that support their effective implementation.

There are a number of reasons for this:

- We have hardly helped ourselves over the last few years with the proliferation of different languages that we have employed to describe different ways of enabling people to have choice and control over their care and support. Personalisation may now be common parlance, but people can still mean very different things by it. Self-directed support similarly, and the concepts and differences between personal budgets, direct payments, personal health budgets, managed budgets and ISFs (the list could go on) are less than clear to most people. We have created an industry of jargon, and not for the first time, while seeking to make some fairly profound changes to the culture and practice of care. The consequences have been more than linguistically significant as debates over terminology have arguably contributed to a systemic inertia around practical ideas that could be far more broadly applied to universal benefit. ISFs are one such idea.

- Beyond the language we use, there has been a lack of clarity about exactly what we are referring to when we talk about ISFs. This has some specific elements – such as my own unhelpful contribution to the debate when I referred to ISFs in an early paper for the Department of Health as three way "contracts" between the commissioning agency, the provider and the person needing care and support. They are in fact nothing of the sort, and are rarely "contracts" of any kind, unless the ISF is administered for a direct payment holder. And therein lies the deeper problem, that there are so many permutations and different uses for ISFs that it can be counterproductive to pin them down beyond some basic principles. Greater conceptual clarity could serve to limit their application...which is all well and good, but doesn't help when you are trying to advocate for them!

The point here is that ISFs are an idea, and a practical set of principles and practices that can help to deliver more personalised care and support in any setting, from supported living, to homecare, to residential and nursing. They will look different in each instance, naturally. And the process of implementing them will be different depending on whether the principles are applied to a block contracted service, or to the task of setting a service up from scratch around an individual. Are you still following me? It will get clearer, I promise!

- Linked to this, even where we have got it clear in our minds how taking an ISF approach could be really helpful, it has often not been obvious whose job it is to be getting on with actually doing it. Is it for the commissioner to set the framework and initiate the shift while providers sit and wait? Is it for the provider to take the initiative and start working differently within their existing services, regardless of commissioning involvement? Or is it for the person with the care and support needs to demand a different type of service and a different relationship with their provider? That it is all of these things is testament to the strength and flexibility of the idea, but it can and has led to a good deal of sitting on hands waiting for the lead to be taken by somebody!

- Finally, we have arguably been less clear than we could have been about the intended outcomes and benefits. And let's face it, without a very strong case behind it, any idea that needs effort to realise will find it hard to get off the drawing board in the current environment.

So, what is the case for ISFs? I think this falls into three areas: improving people's experience and satisfaction with care, designing more cost effective solutions and, most importantly, delivering better outcomes for people.

Improving experience and satisfaction

The main driver behind ISFs, an idea that actually predates self-directed support, has been to enable people to make choices and take control of how services support them to live their lives. In more recent times ISFs have also been about trying to bridge the gap between the experience of people using direct payments and those who don't, as managed budget options have tended to provide a lesser degree of choice and control than they can and should.

This is important because people's experience of being in control and of being able to choose the way services work with them is profoundly transformational, yet traditional models of commissioning and service delivery have rarely done this well. Service outputs have often been tightly defined and a culture that encourages rigidity rather than flexibility has been commonplace, with very little thought given to empowering the person in the middle to shape their service and become less, not more, dependent. There are clear linkages also between people's experience of choice and control and their satisfaction levels. The national personal budgets survey published by Think Local Act Personal in 2013 makes it clear that those who feel more in control of important decisions about their support, have control over the process of developing their care and support plan and are able to choose the people who work with them generally have a better experience. We know that not everyone will want or be able to take a direct payment, so it is important that we find ways of extending the idea and experience of choice and control to everyone, and ISFs are most certainly part of the solution.

When ISFs are done well (and like anything there are certainly plenty of ways of doing them badly!) they can change the nature of the relationship between provider and the person being supported. They can underpin a major shift in culture and practice towards genuine personalisation and they can provide a practical set of tools for making managed budgets more meaningful. They can improve people's experience of and satisfaction with care and support – and that is something we should all be interested in!

Designing more cost effective solutions

In the current environment however, improved experience and satisfaction levels may not be enough to warrant the effort needed. With prolonged pressure on public finances inevitably come strategies – good and bad – for managing budget reductions. In the worst instances this can involve quick and crude salami slicing, imposed without any real engagement and agreement between commissioners, providers and people, carers and families about how the saving can be made. In better instances, very difficult decisions are made together about how a service can work differently and change is managed through in partnership. None of this is easy and arguably the current challenges for the sector are uniquely acute. It will not be possible to just do less of the same more cheaply, which makes it critically important that service redesign as a collaborative and shared endeavor is seen as part of the solution.

Integral to the ISF process is the unpicking of aggregate contracts, particularly in shared accommodation, and the rebuilding of support around the specific needs and preferences of each individual. This discipline presents a positive challenge to the cost base of services, can unearth historical anomalies and often provides numerous opportunities to think and do things differently. This won't always mean savings, but it often does. When done well, the ISF process also involves the application of the principles and practice of 'just enough support,' which involves looking at people's support in the round, with paid support as only one part of the solution and thinking creatively, including giving active consideration to the use of assistive technology and informal and community based support in each instance. While the formal evidence base for savings from ISFs is still limited, there are plenty of instances where the approach seems to be delivering the ideal scenario of cost reductions and improving outcomes. Alternative Futures Group's work with Knowsley (shortly to be written up) is one such case, where savings of around 15 per cent have been delivered at the same time as enabling people to have more tailored support.

Delivering better outcomes

This book is packed full of stories that illustrate the outcomes for people that can result from deploying an ISF model. It focuses on the outstanding work that has been done at Bruce Lodge, a large care home for people with dementia now arranged as 43 separate ISFs, with every resident able to control a number of hours of support that are set aside for them to do the things they want, when and where they want. But versions of these stories are available for all sorts of different environments, from the model a number of providers are rolling out across all their supported living services, to the groundbreaking work that has been done more recently to translate ISFs into something that works for people receiving care at home. Delivering better outcomes is at the heart of all of these stories, and it is at the heart of this book.

To draw out one of the many stories you will read about in these pages, nothing says it better than Winifred's story:

Winifred's daughters and the team at Bruce Lodge recognised Winifred was feeling lost at times and so they focused on her gifts and understanding when were the times her wellbeing was at its best. This led to the resounding answer that Winifred was happiest when helping Beryl, the housekeeper, so Winifred's ISF has been about structuring her time so that she can spend more of it with Beryl.

It has now become simply the way Winifred spends each day, carrying out the household chores with Beryl. She can be heard singing aloud as she polishes, mops, washes up and carries out the chores she did so routinely in her own home before she moved here. Winifred's new relationship with Beryl and extra responsibility has had an extraordinary effect on her happiness and wellbeing. Maureen and Bernie, Winifred's daughters, have noticed the change – she is happier, chatting more, using fuller sentences, sleeping better and is generally 'more alive'.

Maureen goes on to say:

> *The difference is astounding; mum was a housewife, a practical person who spent her life caring for her five children and our father, who died 20 years ago. Her desire to care for people was never blunted but the ability to do so was robbed from her and that left her very frustrated. These chores are helping her connect with other things from her past and are opening up new pathways in her mind. The first thing that we noticed had come back was her language – within a week of working with Beryl she was recalling words much better and introducing me to other people by name, whereas before she didn't know who I was.*

I feel sure that this book will help many more people to bring about these positive changes within services and within people's lives.

Dr Sam Bennett
Programme Director,
Think Local Act Personal

1

Introduction and Getting Started

MARIE

Marie is an unassuming, quietly-spoken, warm and generous woman.

She says, 'My family are everything to me.' Marie lived with her late husband, Frank, in Appleton. Her favourite memories are of working in various offices, her honeymoon in Ireland in 1958 and celebrating her children's birthdays together as a family each year. The important people in Marie's life now are her sons Stefan, who visits often, and Carl, who lives in London, and Marie and Collette, her two nieces.

Marie prefers to spend time in her room surrounded by her family photographs and personal possessions. She likes her privacy rather than communal living, though she always welcomes callers to her room to have a chat with her.

Marie has always been a devout Catholic, and she and her husband met in the Catholic Social Club. It was a long time since Marie had been to Mass, and she missed it. Although seeing Tim – the Eucharistic minister who visits the home each week – was a joy, going to Mass was something that was important to Marie and she really wanted to go to Mass each week.

To go back to Mass at St Joseph's Church was clearly the way that Marie wanted to spend her individual time. When it came to choosing someone for her to go with, the obvious match would be someone who was also a devout Catholic, and ideally someone who attended the same church. That person was a staff member called Olivia.

Marie is becoming more involved in the church and getting to know the people there much better. Marie was always a key part of the St Vincent de Paul Society at the church, and she'd really love to get involved again: Olivia is working on this. There are a number of people at church Marie is getting to know well and with whom she thoroughly enjoys spending time.

Staff have learned more about what good support looks like for Marie [see Figure 1.1] Marie is a very gentle lady and can be startled by people who speak loudly, or become overwhelmed if people embark on loud or rushed conversations with her. Marie feels the cold, and must be really well wrapped. Even in the summer months she still feels cold, so staff now always ensure Marie is wearing socks or stockings, and know that if it is chilly, an extra jumper will always go down well.

Going to Mass regularly has made a huge difference to Marie. She says, 'It's wonderful to be able to say my prayers, kneeling before the cross.' She feels reconnected with her faith and her community, and has a staff member with whom she can talk about her faith and the church.

'Come back to me when you have done this for 20 people'

This was David Behan's (then the Director General for Adult Social Care) challenge to Helen Sanderson when she launched a book[1] at the National Children and Adult Services Conference in London in November 2010 in which Steve Scown and Helen describe how they worked with six people in a residential care home to introduce Individual Service Funds (ISFs) so that people could have more choice and control in their lives. David Behan's challenge was for us to go from 6 to 20, and to see if we could make ISFs work for people living with dementia.

We all know that people living with dementia must be treated with dignity and respect, and that good services provide person-centred care. We also know that in good care homes staff spend time learning about the person's life history.

Personalisation builds on person-centred care. Personalisation means that as well as treating people with dignity and respect, we must also strongly focus on helping people direct their own service and have as much choice and control in their life as possible. Instead of fitting people into existing services it means designing their service around them. People get the support they want and need, when they want it, in the way that they want it, at the time they want, delivered by the person they want.

---

1   Scown, S. and Sandseron, H. (2011) *Making it Personal for Everyone: From Block Contracts towards Individual Service Funds.* Stockport: HSA.

What is important to Marie

- Her sons, Stefan who visits often, and Carl who lives in London and travels up to visit as regularly as possible.
- Marie Kennedy and her sister Colette – Marie's nieces who visit regularly.
- Her Roman Catholic faith. Going to mass at St. Joseph's every Sunday
- Seeing Tim, the Eucharistic minister, each week.
- Manchester City – Marie loves talking about the club!
- Marie loves mealtimes – cereal and a full cooked breakfast is favourite!
- Drinks of juice often and a snack – Marie has a sweet tooth!
- To have someone sit and read poetry to her. Marie loves poetry, she had an anthology published in 2001.
- That people take the time to talk with her.
- Watching what is happening around the home and chatting with others who live and work here.
- Spending time and having conversations with Doreen, who lives here.
- Marie must not be cold!
- Patience Strong poetry books are very special to Marie, read them with her often
- Cutting Patience Strong verse out of any magazines such as People's Friend and collating them in a scrap book
- Going out to cafes for a drink and watching the outside world go by, she is very mindful and will comment on how beautiful the colour of the traffic lights are.
- Fresh flowers are a must!
- Having her hair nicely plaited

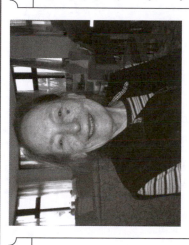

Marie

What those who know Marie best say they like and admire about her

A very friendly lady

Gentle – never a bad word to say about anybody

A quick thinker

A real 'doer'

How we can best support Marie

- Know that Marie feels the cold, always check out with her if she is warm enough.
- Marie must always use her frame when walking.
- Be aware that Marie has diabetes – see care plan for detail.
- Marie is a very quiet, unassuming lady but know that she loves conversation, always take the time to chat with her.
- The chain Marie wore around her neck has been lost, she has had it for many years and never took it off, help her find it
- Always ensure Marie is wearing socks or stockings – she really feels the cold. If it is chilly help her put an extra jumper or cardy on
- If Marie is going out walking any distance it is good to take a wheelchair in case she needs it.
- Involve Marie in conversation often, she is such a quiet gentle lady she can easily become invisible – religion, poetry and crafts are favourite topics
- Know that Marie struggles sometimes to find the bathroom – especially first thing in the morning, ask her regularly if she wants to go to the bathroom – if she says no then she doesn't.
- Know that Marie doesn't wear make up and wouldn't appreciate having her nails painted – be aware however she does enjoy pampering & looking nice
- Always leave a jumper at the bottom of Marie's bed in case she feels cold in the night, she will really appreciate this
- Always speak gently to Marie, she is a very gentle lady and can find loud voices overwhelming
- Know that Marie must blow her nose after using the toilet, ensure she always has plenty of tissues
- Marie's walking frame and slippers must always be left within easy reach when she goes to bed, the bathroom light must be kept on.

Figure 1.1 Marie's one-page profile

One way to deliver personalisation is through personal budgets, where people have a budget to buy their services themselves. The government is piloting personal budgets in residential care homes so that in the future ISFs (where people use their personal budget to buy their support from a service provider) will be how care homes are funded.

Some people asked whether personalisation in care homes is really possible. Can we offer more personalised support to people who live in residential care, or should we, as some have suggested, be putting all efforts instead into closing congregate living?

Here is a challenge: how far can we go in offering a more personalised service within a care home? Can we still apply the same principles of good practice when using ISFs[2] in a care home setting?

What an Individual Service Fund means in practice

- *What*: I can use my hours or budget flexibly and can choose what I am supported with.

- *Where*: I am supported where it makes sense for me, at home and out and about.

- *Who*: I choose who I want to support me, my support worker knows me and I know them.

- *When*: I get support on the days and at the times that are right for me.

- *How*: I choose how I am supported and my support workers know what is important to me.

- *Co-production*: I am fully involved in decisions about my own support and about how the wider service develops.

---

2   Developed by Groundswell Partnership in Sanderson, H., Bennett, S., Stockton, S. and Lewis, J. (2012) *Choice and Control for All: The Role of Individual Service Funds in Delivering Fully Personalised Care and Support*. London: Groundswell.

How can we make Individual Service Funds work in residential care?

We wanted to see if this could work at two levels: first, to introduce the principles of ISFs and make sure that each person had their own allocation of time or money; and second, to make sure that everyone had a truly personalised service, was seen and treated as an individual and could direct their own support as much as possible.

Helen lives in Stockport, so her first thought was to see if we could find a way to deliver ISFs for people living with dementia in a care home in Stockport. She had met Terry Dafter, the Director of Adult Social Care, a few times, so she emailed him. She met up with Joan Beresford, then Head of Older People's Services, Mark Warren (Head of Social Work), Paul Oakley (Workforce Development) and Chris Waddleton (Contracts and Monitoring), who were all enthusiastic and keen to start.

Within three months, we had a project in place, and all the care home providers in Stockport Council had been invited to be part of it. Borough Care Ltd came forward.

Helen says:

> I clearly remember the first time I met Lisa, the manager of Bruce Lodge. We had a two-hour meeting to introduce the project to all of the managers from across Borough Care. I did a presentation on what we had learned from Making it Personal. Lisa sat there with her arms folded across her chest. I remember thinking that it would be a challenge if Lisa was the manager they selected to be involved.

Bruce Lodge was selected as the care home for us to work with.

Lisa started work as a volunteer 26 years ago, then became a care assistant, then senior care assistant and is now the manager at Bruce Lodge. She said:

> I was really not sure that what Helen was talking about was possible. We were already stretched, already trying our hardest to get all the tasks that we had to do done. How could we do more without more staff? I admit that I was sceptical at the start, but willing to give it a go.

The leadership team

We had now established a partnership between Stockport Council, Borough Care Ltd and Helen Sanderson Associates (HSA).

Here was our task:

- For each person living with dementia at Bruce Lodge to direct their own support on a day-to-day basis, by staff knowing what mattered to each person (what was important to them) and what good support looked like, so that they could consistently deliver this.

- For each person to have a monthly allocation of time that they could determine how to use, with the one-to-one support of a staff member they chose.

Our challenge was to do this without any increase in resources at Bruce Lodge. The only additional support was three half-days of training, and ten days of Gill Bailey from HSA's time to coach and support Lisa and the staff.

We put together a leadership team from Borough Care Ltd, HSA and Stockport Local Authority. The team met every month. For the first four months we met for a whole day to fully establish the project, then we met for half days each month to look at the learning, to problem-solve and to monitor progress. Overall we had 14 meetings between April 2012 and July 2013.

The membership of the leadership team was:

- HSA – Helen facilitating the project and leadership team meetings; Gill providing the direct support to Bruce Lodge

- Borough Care Ltd
  - Kathy Farmer, CEO
  - Ines Kirby, Deputy CEO
  - Lisa Bruce, Manager of Bruce Lodge
  - Seniors – for specific meetings

- Stockport Council
  - Joan Beresford, Integrated Commissioner

- ○ Mark Warren, Service Manager in Older People's Services

- ○ Paul Oakley, Workforce Lead

- ○ Chris Waddleton, Contracts and Compliance

- ○ Stella Clare, Quality Lead

- ○ Sue Griffiths and Patsy Wyles, Communications Team members.

Stockport Council saw this as a pilot to explore what was possible and how to make it happen. Therefore, their staff on the leadership team had a present and a future focus – how to support the current project, and the implications for extending it throughout the area.

- Paul, the workforce lead, was there to support the process and to learn how the workforce would need to be supported in the future, in order to implement personalisation and ISFs in care homes.

- Chris, the contracts lead, was there to support the process and see what adjustments may be needed to contracts and compliance to enable ISFs to be delivered in the future.

- Sue and Patsy shared the communications role. They were there to support the sharing of information across the council and with other stakeholders.

We thought about how we could make sure that people living with dementia and their families could be involved. Although Stockport has a strong commitment to co-production, this has usually involved working in partnership with family-led organisations, self-advocacy or advocacy organisations. There is no equivalent in Stockport for people living with dementia. We made sure we had lots of ways to hear the views of family members (see Chapter 2) and we acted on these through the leadership team. The views of people living with dementia entirely directed the third phase of our work, and we describe this in Chapter 8.

How we worked together

You may have had the experience of sitting on a steering group. Typically, the group takes reports from the people they are 'steering' and makes recommendations as the project progresses. We wanted this to be a very different kind of group, who worked together in a person-centred way and led the project from its centre.

Person-centred teams have a culture of trust, empowerment and accountability,[3] and as a leadership team we tried to develop this culture within the way we worked. This is what we did:[4]

1. Opening and closing rounds

We started each meeting by asking everyone to share, in turn, something that was going well for them at work (about this project where possible), and at home. This meant that we started each meeting positively, and we got to know each other better by hearing something about people's lives outside work. A great by-product of the opening rounds was that we learned that Chris was a lay minister, and we used his expertise when we looked at working with faith communities, described in Chapter 7.

We closed meetings with a round where we asked each person to share something that they appreciated about the meeting. This helped us all to reflect on the progress we were making together.

We also used rounds at different times in our meetings. This was particularly important given the breadth of roles, and the span of seniority from seniors to CEO and commissioner. Everyone's view was important, but not everyone felt confident speaking up: rounds were a great way to ensure we had everyone's contribution to each discussion.

2. Outcome-based agendas

The agenda stated the outcomes that we wanted to achieve for each agenda item, the time for each section, and how people could

---

3   Sanderson, H. and Lepkowsky, M.B. (2014) *Person-Centred Teams.* Stockport: HSA.

4   These are taken from HSA's Positive and Productive Meetings. To learn more about this process go to www.helensandersonassociates.co.uk.

prepare for the meeting. You can see an example of one of our agendas in the Appendix.

3. One-page profiles: Leading by example

Members of the leadership team attended the training on one-page profiles with staff from Bruce Lodge, and did their own one-page profiles. We shared these within the leadership team, so that we could get to know each other more, as well as have the experience of doing our own one-page profile. This gave the leadership team greater insight into what we were expecting of the staff.

4. Using person-centred practices

We used person-centred practices within our meetings and in the way that we worked together, for example:

- We looked at what was *working and not working from different perspectives* in our meetings and used this as the basis of celebration and problem solving.

- We developed a shared *doughnut* (a person-centred thinking tool),[5] which clarified expectations of different people in the way one-page profiles for staff were being developed.

5. Clear purpose and a shared understanding of success

As you will read in Chapter 2, one of our first decisions was what success looked like from each of our perspectives. What would we see happening for people living at Bruce Lodge? What difference did we want to make in the way that staff worked? What would it mean for each of our organisations? This meant that we stayed focused on success in each of our meetings.

---

5   To learn more about the doughnut go to www.helensandersonassociates.co.uk.

6. Clear roles and expectations

We spent time clarifying both what success looked like for each of the three partners, and what their responsibilities were in delivering this. There were no passengers on the leadership team!

Chris and Paul's involvement was primarily to look at the future implications around contracts and human resources. Typically in steering groups, people with roles like this comment on what is happening without being directly involved. We wanted them to have a direct role as well. So Chris and Paul took it in turns, week by week, to phone Lisa and to talk to her about how the project was going. They then fed that information back into the leadership team. Chris and Paul therefore had a support role through regular contact with Lisa.

Obviously Lisa's manager, Ines, had a crucial role in supporting Lisa to implement the project, which she did through her supervision of Lisa.

Gill's role was to coach and support Lisa and the staff on the site to give them the tools and understanding they needed to make the project happen.

7. Shared accountability

In addition to the detailed list of actions developed at each meeting, which we revisited at the next meeting, we had our dashboard as a standing agenda item. This was a clear record of how we were doing, and it ensured we were accountable to each other for progress.

Before we began

Our diaries were busy, and the earliest day that everyone could make was in April. We decided to get started in an earlier initial meeting of part of the team for a couple of hours in March. At this meeting we did important preparatory work around resource allocation, and organised gathering baseline data and agreeing standards for one-page profiles.

a) Resource allocation: How much time could each person have?

We did not try to deconstruct the block contract into individual budget allocations. We saw this as important in the future, but took the pragmatic decision to have a budget of hours rather than money at the outset. Later we disaggregated the activities budget into individual budgets, in addition to personal hours.

Practically, we did not think that any less than two hours would be worth doing. We asked Borough Care to commit to what was practical and possible within their existing staff allocation. This led to agreeing an individual 'budget' of two hours a month per person.

When we presented this at a conference in 2012, there were audible gasps. The majority of participants were from other service sectors, in particular those supporting people with learning disabilities. There was disbelief that the allocation was so small, and we heard comments like, 'Only two hours a month? What difference could that make?' and 'Is that even worth doing?' Sharing what we were doing with colleagues who support people living with dementia created a different reaction: 'Two hours a month – how have you managed that without extra funding?'

We reminded people that we were trying to do two things: to introduce individual time *and* more personalised support. We had to start with where we were and what was possible, and go from there. We've found time and time again that we make real progress when we follow the words of Arthur Ashe, the US tennis player and social activist: 'Start where you are. Use what you have. Do what you can.'

b) Baseline data: Where are we starting from?

We started by evaluating what the service was like at the time of the first meeting, so that we could measure what changed. We used two observational tools: Dementia Care Mapping (DCM), and the Quality of Interactions Schedule (QUIS), along with Progress for Providers: Checking your progress in delivering personalised services (see Chapter 9).

c) Agreeing standards for one-page profiles

We already knew that we would need to develop one-page profiles for people living at Bruce Lodge and the staff who worked there. We learnt from *Making it Personal* how important it is to clarify what one-page profiles are, how they will be used and what the standards are. We asked Gill to do this with Ines and Lisa before the first leadership team meeting. You can find the one-page profile standards in the Appendix.

Chapter summary: Setting up the leadership team for success

Setting up the team helped us to see the possible scope of the project, where we were starting from and what we would need to deliver it. We established how we would make sure that everyone affected by the project was fully involved, and one way we did this was to allocate active roles to every team member.

In the next chapter, we look at how we decided what success would look like for our team, how we would measure it and how we would tell everyone what we were doing.

2

Plans and Processes

ELLEN

Ellen was 98, and the first person to have what the staff called 'personalisation time'. Sadly she died six months later. She had two sons, Stan and Roy, who visited her. It was always important to Ellen that she sat near the window or patio door where she could look out. She would count the planes that flew over and would tell you exactly how many there had been. She loved watching the squirrels playing about in the garden. Ellen watched who was coming and going around the home and always needed to be supported to sit where she could keep an eye on what was happening both inside and outdoors!

If you went to Bruce Lodge, you were likely to hear Ellen because she was a wonderful singer and often sang Christmas carols in the summer to raise a few smiles! She took great pride in her appearance and loved to have her hair tied up or plaited with a bobble. A big Manchester United fan, Ellen also enjoyed watching horse racing.

What was not working for Ellen was that she was spending a lot of time in her room and was not going out very much.

Ellen said:

I would love to go out to a café for a brew and a cake, or the park watching people, the dogs and the children playing. Then reading the war memorial on the tree in the park for the animals lost or who were a part of the war effort.

Ellen used her personalisation time to get out and about. She loved going to the war memorial and out for a brew and cake with a staff member who shared her love of animals. Staff used her one-page profile on a daily basis and made sure she was sat next to the door or the patio window to count the planes, and watch the birds. They talked to her about the latest Manchester United games, and betting on the horses. She was supported consistently, and talked about her interests with staff.

What is important to Ellen

- Saying her prayers to herself before she goes to sleep. Ellen believes in God.
- Stan & Roy, Ellen's two sons who visit often.
- Ellen must sit near the window or patio door where she can look out. She counts the planes which fly over & will tell you exactly how many.
- Watching the squirrels playing about in the garden.
- Ellen loves birds & will tell you she would feed the robins all day.
- Ellen watches who is coming and going around the home and must always be supported to sit where she can keep an eye on what's happening both inside & outdoors!
- Singing! Ellen is a wonderful singer and often sings Christmas carols in the Summer to raise a few smiles!
- Ellen thoroughly enjoys her bed and a nap during the day suits her just fine.
- Ellen takes pride in her appearance and the clothes she wears.
- Chocolates! Milk, soft ones are her favourite.
- To have her hair tied up or plaited and a bobble in.
- To be told how lovely she looks & chat about her clothes with her.
- Watching horse racing is a love of Ellen's and football – Manchester United are her favourite.

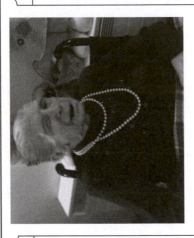

Ellen

What those who know Ellen best say they like and admire about her

A huge character

Salt of the earth

A grand woman and very wise

Wicked sense of humour and her winks

Straightforward – says it as it is and stands her ground

Very happy go lucky lady – an inspiration to others

How we can best support Ellen

- Ellen must be kept warm at all times.
- Always support Ellen to sit where she can look out of the window.
- Ellen loves birds – chat with her about the birds in the garden and when it is warm help her into the garden to feed the birds. Ellen must always be wrapped up well even if it feels warm outside – she is prone to chest infections & bouts of pneumonia.
- Know that Ellen will have lots of little naps during the day – she says there's nothing wrong with that at 98!
- If Ellen tells you she wants something – for example to go to bed for a nap, you should acknowledge & act on her request.
- Know that Ellen will sometimes shout at you & say she wants to die. She will usually feel better after a cup of tea and a cream biscuit. Know that chatting to her about Stan and Roy or looking out at the birds & squirrels helps too.
- Know that Ellen is in control & we have to conform with her!
- When Ellen is very vocal and upset know that what works best for her is some time to herself.

Figure 2.1 Ellen's one-page profile

Thinking about success and communication

Most projects begin with a project plan. We made three decisions at our first leadership team meeting before we started on the project plan. We decided:

- what success would mean from different perspectives

- how we were going to measure whether we were being successful or not, and how we were going to learn from other people about how the project was going

- how we were going to communicate what we were doing, both internally (within each of the three partner organisations) and externally.

We were clear about our overall purpose – implementing personalisation and exploring ISFs. Now we wanted to drill down further and think about what we would see in people's lives, or hear them saying, if we were successful.

We also wanted to find a way easily to share what we were doing with everyone (without necessarily using the terms Individual Service Funds or personalisation).

Taking this approach helped us to clarify what we hoped to see, and to recognise that success would mean different things for different people. We wanted a win-win-win-win: to work together to make a positive difference to people who live at Bruce Lodge, to staff, to Borough Care and to Stockport Council. Being able to clearly describe this would also really help with how we communicated what we were trying to do to the different audiences and stakeholder groups that our partnership reflects.

We developed this as a one-page strategy – an at-a-glance summary of what we wanted to achieve, who for, and how. You can see this in the Appendix.

Success from different perspectives
Success for the people living at Bruce Lodge

We started by focusing on what success would look like to the people who live at Bruce Lodge. We developed 'I' statements to express the changes we wanted people to feel and experience.

Although in reality people may not be able to express what they want in these words, the statements reflect the sentiments of what they wanted and so reflect the principles that we are working to with ISFs.

For people living at Bruce Lodge we thought that we would be successful when they were able to experience the following:

- *I'm supported by people who know me, and act on what matters to me now and on how I want to be supported.* To deliver a truly personalised service people needed to be known and treated as individuals, in a way that reflected both what mattered to them, and how they wanted to be supported.

- *I'm listened to and heard, and supported to make choices and decisions.* We wanted people to be involved in their day-to-day life in a way that worked for them. We wanted people to be listened to and heard, and to make choices and decisions, as this reflects the key principles around personalisation.

- *I have individual time each month and choose what I do and who supports me.* Because we wanted to implement ISFs, we needed a success statement that reflected this: people having individual time each month, and choosing what they do and who supported them was fundamental to this.

These statements closely link to the National Dementia Declaration. This helped us feel confident that this is what people themselves would want.

The National Dementia Declaration[1] says:

1. I have personal choice and control or influence over decisions about me.

2. I know that services are designed around me and my needs.

3. I have support that helps me live my life.

4. I have the knowledge and know-how to get what I need.

---

1   National Dementia Declaration (2014) Dementia Action Alliance (UK). Available at www.dementiaaction.org.uk/nationaldementiadeclaration, accessed on 23 June 2014.

5. I live in an enabling and supportive environment where I feel valued and understood.

6. I have a sense of belonging and of being a valued part of family, community and civic life.

7. I know there is research going on which delivers a better life for me now and hope for the future.

Success for the staff at Bruce Lodge

We also wanted to make a positive difference in the lives of staff. We wanted staff to feel listened to, and to be able to contribute to the lives of the people they supported, and to the home and the success of the organisation. We wanted staff to feel that their hobbies and interests were matched to how people living at Bruce Lodge wanted to spend their individual time. And we wanted staff to have a greater sense of job satisfaction from doing a great job and supporting people in a person-centred way on a day-to-day basis.

There are lots of initiatives and projects aspiring to change the lives of people with dementia. We think that it is crucial to change the staff's experience as part of this. Nationally, we have been learning that if you want to implement personalisation and person-centred practices, you have to be person-centred with staff as well as the people they support. Of course, we wanted staff to feel listened to, able to contribute, supported in a way that mattered to them and satisfied in their work. But we wanted to go even further and take into account each person as a whole, matching their hobbies and interests to individuals living in the home.

So those were the first two key areas we wanted to look at: what success would mean for people living at Bruce Lodge, and what success would mean for staff.

Success for Borough Care

What was in this for Borough Care? Although a letter from Chris Waddleton went to every care home provider in the area, only Borough Care came forward and expressed an interest. We wanted to be clear about what success meant to them as a business. Having

Kathy, Ines and Lisa in the room meant that we could ask them directly. They said that success for them was:

- to be seen and feel like they're delivering a person-centred service that people have confidence in and want to buy

- to demonstrate and share good practice in delivering personalised services for people living with dementia in care homes. This meant moving beyond person-centred care to being known and seen as an organisation that delivers personalised services.

- to know and act on what's working and not working for people using services, and working in our services. This meant that both people receiving services and staff were directly influencing the future direction of the service.

Success for Stockport Council

And finally for Stockport Council. On the team we had Joan, Mark, Paul and Chris who could tell us directly how the council hoped to benefit. Stockport Council wanted:

- to know that they were commissioning personalised services that were safe and offered real choice for people living with dementia in Stockport

- to be working in active partnership with providers to deliver personalised services for people living in care homes, and to be able to share what they were learning locally, regionally and nationally.

Delivering and measuring success

Describing what success would look like gave us the first, top level of our one-page strategy. A one-page strategy has three different levels. The first level is what success means from different perspectives, and for this project that was from the perspectives of people living at Bruce Lodge, staff at Bruce Lodge, Borough Care and Stockport Council. The next level is how we would deliver this – the different processes and practices that we were planning to use to deliver success. The third level described how we were going to measure how successful we were being.

We know that what gets measured gets done, so to complete the one-page strategy we needed to think about what we were going to measure and demonstrate change. The following tables summarise each success statement, how we wanted to deliver it and how we were going to measure whether we had been successful or not.

Table 2.1 People living at Bruce Lodge

Success statement	How we could deliver this, and rationale	What we could measure
I am supported by people who know me, and act on what matters to me now, for my future and how I want to be supported.	One-page profiles describe what matters to the person and how they want to be supported; therefore each individual having a one-page profile was important. We also needed to learn what people wanted in the future, so used 'If I could, I would' in the one-page profile meetings.	• Number of people with one-page profiles that meet standards, with working/not working • Number of people with communication charts/decision-making agreements • Number of people who have a clear, specified outcome for using their two hours' individual time • Increase in scores from Dementia Care Map
I am listened to and heard, and supported to make choices and decisions.	We heard what is working and not working for each person as part of the one-page profile meetings. By changing what is not working, this demonstrates how we are hearing and acting on what people have told us. Using communication charts and decision-making agreements are ways for staff to understand how to support people to make choices and decisions.	
I have individual time each month and choose what I do and who supports me.	Each person had two hours a month and Lisa suggested a match to the person based on shared interests with staff members.	

Table 2.2 Staff

Success statement	How we could deliver this, and rationale	What we could measure
Our hobbies and interests are matched to how people living at Bruce Lodge want to spend their individual time.	To deliver this we needed to know each staff member's hobbies and interests. Therefore, each staff member needed their own one-page profile.	• Number of staff with one-page profiles that meet standards • Matching staff used for each individual based on how they want to spend their individual two hours • Percentage of learning logs used to capture learning on how people spent their individual time • Increase in scores from Progress for Providers.
We are listened to and able to contribute to the lives of the people we support, the home and success of the organisation.	Using learning logs is one way to hear what staff are learning about the individual. Staff also contributed by using their comments and reflections on what is working and not working about the process, and this was used to co-design the second phase of the programme.	
We get satisfaction from doing a great job and supporting people in a person-centred way on a day-to-day basis, and with their individual hours.	With each individual who lives at Bruce Lodge having a one-page profile, staff will know in detail how to support them; by delivering this they can feel confident that they are doing a good job.	

Table 2.3 The leadership team: Borough Care and Stockport Council

Success statement	How we could deliver this and rationale	What we could measure
We are delivering a person-centred service that people have confidence in, and want to buy.	A person-centred service has to start with knowing what matters to each person and how they want to be supported, therefore everyone having a one-page profile is important.	• Percentage of people living at Bruce Lodge whose individual time is delivered by a key worker. We are looking for staff to be chosen individually and not expecting this to always be the key worker
We demonstrate and share good practice in delivering personalised services for people living with dementia in care homes.	We focused on how we could record what we are learning and share this through our communication strategy.	• Analysis of how the two hours are used per person. We are expecting to see variety, for example, some people having their two hours a month in four half-hour sessions
We know and act on what's working and what's not working for people using and working in our services.	Using 'working and not working' initially in the one-page profile meeting and then regularly through person-centred reviews.	• Percentage of people who use their individual time outside Bruce Lodge. We are looking for a high percentage of people to use their time in the community
		• Range of creative options (versus traditional options) tried to enable people to use their two hours in a way that they want

cont.

Table 2.3 The leadership team: Borough Care and Stockport Council *cont.*

Success statement	How we could deliver this and rationale	What we could measure

We are commissioning personalised services which are safe and offer real choice for the people living with dementia in Stockport.	We demonstrate that people have choice through how they use their individual time, and using communication charts and decision-making agreements. The safest services are the ones that really pay attention to how to support people well (as described on one-page profiles).	• Increase in the scores from Dementia Mapping and Observation Schedule (QUIS)
		
		• Increase in scores from Progress for Providers
		
		• Percentage of actions achieved from Dementia Mapping recommendations
		
		• Number of places/ways where information about this has been shared
		  ○ Internally
		  ○ Externally (regionally and nationally)

We share what we are learning locally, regionally and nationally.	The communication strategy needed to include local and national sharing of learning.	

More than numbers

One of Helen's favourite ways of thinking about quality comes from the work of Mark Friedman.[2] He suggests that in thinking about quality you need to focus on three questions:

- What are we doing?

- Are we doing enough?

- Is it making a difference?

---

2   Friedman, M. (2005) *Trying Hard is not Good Enough: How to Produce Measurable Improvements for Customers and Communities.* Victoria, BC: Trafford.

Our one-page strategy clearly describes what we want to achieve (success from different perspectives), how we are doing it (how we deliver success) and how much we are doing (are we doing enough?), but these refer to what we are doing (processes), not what difference it makes.

We needed to do more than count our person-centred processes, so here are the ways we used to learn more about whether what we were doing was making a difference:

- Dementia Care Mapping

- QUIS

- comments and reflections from families, staff and professionals

- what people said was working and not working for them through person-centred reviews (Working Together for Change)

- stories.

We have threaded some of these stories of change throughout the book. In Chapter 8 we share what we learned from what people said was working and not working for them, and in Chapter 9 we talk about what difference the Dementia Care Map indicated.

We wanted to be really rigorous in knowing how well we were doing, and being accountable, so we kept track of our numbers though a dashboard at the beginning of every leadership team meeting. When we started in June we decided to look at the number of people who had a one-page profile and what was working/not working, and the number of people with communication charts and decision-making agreements. We gathered this information before each meeting, and then we'd look at it as part of the meeting, as a standing agenda item. For staff we looked at the total number of staff one-page profiles, and the number of completed learning logs. For each of those indicators we would have a number, and we'd expect to see that number increasing month on month. You can see how we structured our dashboard in the Appendix.

Communication strategy

The third decision that we made, after what success looked like and how to measure it, was how to communicate what we were doing and learning. We knew that in order to make a significant change in the way that we were working at Bruce Lodge we needed to make sure we had a wide variety of ways to keep everybody informed and involved.

The most important people to communicate with were the individuals, relatives and staff. In addition, each of the three organisations in the partnership – Borough Care Ltd, Stockport Council and ourselves – had key stakeholders that they needed to keep informed. To develop the communication strategy we mapped out the key stakeholders from each organisation's perspective, and decided the best ways to keep them informed, how often, and who would be responsible for making that happen. We added some of this information to the dashboard.

Here are some examples:

Families and staff at Bruce Lodge

- There was a monthly meeting of families and service users. The work that we were doing was put as an agenda item at the meeting to make sure family members and residents knew about the project and had opportunities to ask questions.

- Borough Care updated their information pack to let new and existing residents and families know about the project and why we were doing one-page profiles and what they looked like.

- We used comments cards to tell people about the project and let them know how they could give us their feedback and tell us how it was going. We also designed some information sheets to go on the noticeboard for people to look at. We put the post box for the comments cards next to the noticeboard so people could both find out about what we were doing and post their comments.

- Borough Care let people know about the project through their newsletter, *Magnolia Press*. This is part of the rolling news about Borough Care that they cascade to staff to keep them up to date.

Adult social care managers and staff

Joan made sure that our project was on the agenda of the senior management team for adult social care on a quarterly basis, so that senior managers could stay up to date with the developments. The best way to keep the rest of the adult social care staff involved and knowledgeable was through the Care Knowledge Portal, which is part of the internal website. Video blogs have been found very successful for staff, so we decided to do a monthly video blog, which included interviewing the key managers who were involved, as well as sharing stories about what this meant for people living at Bruce Lodge.

Other care homes

There are regular meetings bringing all care home providers together. We decided that the September meeting – which was the first one after the project team began to meet – would be an opportunity for Gill and Kerri, the deputy manager, to talk about what they were doing and how it was going.

HSA took responsibility for sharing what we were doing and learning nationally, so we had a monthly blog about the project on the HSA website, tweets and Facebook updates.

Chapter summary: Defining success and telling people about the project

Having set up our team, and knowing that we wanted to use personalisation and ISFs to give people with dementia better lives, we needed to decide how we would know if our work was succeeding.

We looked at success from the perspective of everyone involved in the project: primarily the people living at Bruce Lodge and the staff caring for them, but also Borough Care and Stockport Council.

We then described how we would deliver success, and how we would measure it. Finally, we set up ways for us to keep everyone involved in the project up to date with what we were doing, and to tell the wider world too.

In the next chapter, we look at the one-page profiles that every staff member created, and why they were so important.

3

Starting with Staff One-Page Profiles

KAREN

I'm Karen Boyd, and I'm on the senior team here at Bruce Lodge. I transferred from a different role in Borough Care, and I've been here for five years now, since Bruce Lodge opened. I've worked in care since I was 16. It's my vocation and I've done it forever. I've done all sorts of care, from residential to nursing care. Working with people with dementia is very challenging but very rewarding.

The one-page profile was introduced probably about ten months ago and I have personally found it to be really good for us as staff. Some staff were transferred from different homes and have worked here for eight to ten years. We really didn't know much about some people – for example, we didn't know they have children, or that they like going out over the weekends. It was really interesting to learn that people have a life outside of work.

The one-page profiles told us the things we have in common, and then we're matched to people and them to us. We found we had more interesting things to talk about than we would have before.

The biggest change I've seen since the one-page profiles is staff now spend more time together. Some people used to have their breaks separately, and may sit alone in a room. But since we introduced the one-page profiles, more people have gotten together and gone in the staff room. Some people were shyer than others, so it's brought people out as individuals a more.

We work better as a team now because we all have different ways of working, and the one-page profiles have helped us to recognise how to support each other really well at work.

But I found my [personal] one-page profile [see Figure 3.1] quite difficult to do at first because you don't like to write about yourself and you don't know your qualities. We had group meetings (in groups of eight I think) where we passed a piece of paper around. Everybody wrote something that they appreciated about the other staff. It was really good because you learned that people appreciate the things you do. Not everybody says it to you, and you can't say it yourself, so it was good for us.

A few things that were said about me: 'Karen is bubbly and funny, caring, she's a good person to work with, and gets the job done well.' It's all about teamwork, and the one-page profiles have really helped.

Why start with staff one-page profiles?

We had both pragmatic and philosophical reasons for starting with staff one-page profiles.

Pragmatically, if we were to match people who lived at Bruce Lodge with staff who shared their interests, we needed to know what the staff's interests and hobbies were. This information would be on their one-page profile. In addition, staff learn best about working with one-page profiles by doing their own.

Our philosophical reason was that in order to implement great person-centred practices and personalisation we needed staff to feel that they were supported in a person-centred way as well. If each staff member had a one-page profile, then Lisa, the manager, and the seniors would know what good support looked like for each staff member, and then obviously they'd be in a much better position to be able to provide that support. If every member of staff at Bruce Lodge knew what was important to the others, the team should bond and gel even more closely together.

Four ways to help staff create their one-page profiles

We had four approaches to supporting staff to develop their one-page profiles.

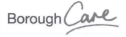 **Karen Boyd**

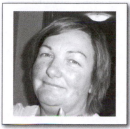

What people like & admire about me
- Supportive
- Kind and caring
- Helpful
- Cheerful and fun
- Hardworking

What's important to me...
- Spending time with my family and my husband
- Visiting my dad two or three times a week
- Ensuring I have a cup of tea when I get up
- Holidays and outings are important to me, I will try anywhere once.
- To keep in touch with my family and friends
- To be prepared and organised at home and in work
- To always be on time as I hate being late
- I like socialising, going to bingo and going to the pub.
- Having a lovely soak bath with candles
- I like cooking, especially Sunday dinners. I also like to eat out at Nandos, Chiquitos and KFC.
- I like going to the cinema to watch chick flicks.
- I like to go to the theatre.

How best to support me...
- I prefer to be part of a team but can manage most tasks on my own
- I like to make a list of tasks to complete so I feel organised
- Please be on time
- I have to take my regular medication on time
- I need to maintain a healthy diet and do some exercise to keep fit

If I could I would like to try...
1) Flower arranging

2) Card making

3) Music and movement

The above should be things that you could try together with one of the people living at Bruce Lodge. For example these could be new hobbies or interests that could be shared such as knitting or attending a football match.

Figure 3.1 Karen's one-page profile

1. We organised training for all staff

There were three repeated half-day training sessions to enable each member of staff to attend. Absolutely every staff member – managers, everybody except the cooks – attended one of the three sessions. The night staff came at the beginning or end of their shift. The leadership team also attended one of these sessions, so that they could learn alongside staff and develop their own one-page profiles. Lisa and Ines had already completed their one-page profiles as part of agreeing the standards with Gill. Their one-page profiles were shared in the training as examples.

2. We established an internal coach

The training uses person-centred thinking tools and exercises to get staff started on their one-page profiles. At the end of the half day, people usually have their one-page profile about 75 per cent complete. After the training, the profile usually needs a little bit of editing and staff need to fill in additional details. We decided that an internal coach, Ian, the training manager at Borough Care, would support the staff to complete their one-page profiles.

3. We organised administrative support

We identified an administrative assistant who would be responsible for making sure all the one-page profiles were typed up into the Bruce Lodge template.

4. We provided some supporting materials

We co-developed these materials with Lisa and Ines, based on a range of examples from working with other organisations. They consisted of one- to two-page summaries explaining what a one-page profile is, how it is developed, how we were going to use it, standards and top tips. We created a template for an individual's one-page profile, and a template for a staff one-page profile (see Figure A2 in the Appendix).

What worked and what didn't work

We found that some of this worked really well, and some of it didn't work out in the way that we had hoped.

Training and materials

Everyone preparing their profiles together, in mixed groups that included members of the leadership team, worked brilliantly. This stage was achieved within two weeks.

Clarity over the purpose and what was expected, as explained in the short, designed materials, helped people to understand the 'why', 'how' and 'what' of one-page profiles. Having Lisa's example to share both demonstrated what the standards looked like in practice, and her commitment and leadership.

The one-page profile templates, with the branding and logo of Borough Care, also showed the organisation's commitment. The quality and thought that had gone into the materials really paid off.

We also learned how important it was that the leadership team walked the walk. Doing the training at the same time and developing their own one-page profiles gave them a much deeper understanding about what we were expecting staff to do in preparing their own profiles and those of the individuals living at Bruce Lodge.

Support and administration

What didn't work as well was asking Ian, the training manager, to be responsible for supporting staff to complete their one-page profiles. The thinking behind this was that we could easily support Ian, as a trainer, to get up to speed with more in-depth knowledge about one-page profiles, and he could draw on his experience in helping people to learn. We also thought that as Ian was not a staff member, we would be contributing a resource to Bruce Lodge and helping Ian learn what it would take to implement personalisation across the organisation.

What we learned was that we had inadvertently made staff one-page profiles 'someone else's business'. Bringing Ian in made it much easier for the senior staff and Lisa to step back from the task and not to see it as their responsibility.

Once we learned this, we decided at the leadership meeting to transfer any further coaching support from Ian to the seniors so that they took responsibility for making sure that the staff one-page profiles were completed, and they met the new Borough Care standards.

The other area that did not work at all was the administration support to type the information that staff developed onto the Borough Care one-page profile template. It was organised but somehow just did not happen. Gill ended up typing up most of the information into the profiles, which was not a good use of her time. This again made finishing the staff one-page profiles 'someone else's business', and took the responsibility for finishing off the one-page profiles with photos away from Lisa and her team.

Ideally, in the future we will use iPads or apps for people to complete their profiles really easily themselves during the training, rather than needing additional typing up afterwards. This is something we are exploring.[1]

One-page profiles: Challenges and opportunities

At the leadership team meeting, when we looked at what had worked and not worked around implementing one-page profiles, Lisa raised the issue of a particular staff member who was very reluctant to share personal information. Does everyone have to have one? 'One staff member has refused to do her profile.' This was one of the 'not working' issues that was brought to the leadership team by Lisa.

We thought together about what was likely to underpin that staff member's refusal, and how we could address it. This extended to how far Borough Care could or would go in making it a requirement that all staff have a one-page profile. Our consensus was that it was crucial that staff felt comfortable sharing information about themselves with people who lived at Bruce Lodge to enable natural conversations to happen and for relationships to develop. We decided that staff could make decisions about how much

---

1   There is a free app to develop a one-page profile at http://miprofile.ca, and there is a helpful resource from the Social Care Institute for Excellence, www.scie. org.uk/publications/elearning/person-centred-practice/resource/2_creating_ profile_0_2.html.

information (and in what detail) they felt comfortable sharing on their one-page profile. But they had to have a one-page profile.

Lisa was surprised that this member of staff was resistant. She knew her as someone who was happy to talk to people who lived at Bruce Lodge about her children and her life, easily chatting, for example, about what she had watched on television the night before. Our conclusion was that it was likely to be a misunderstanding about the purpose of a one-page profile. The action from the leadership meeting was for Lisa to go back and talk to the staff member to make sure she really understood the purpose of her one-page profile, about how comfortable she was sharing that information with people who lived at Bruce Lodge and why she might feel less comfortable about having that recorded. This solved the issue.

It is very important to be able to sell the benefits of one-page profiles to staff, so that they can see what is in it for them. The page of information goes some way to do this. Since then, we have developed a poster with a group of managers describing the benefits of one-page profiles for staff (see Figure 3.2).

Detail and quality

'Some of the one-page profiles don't have enough information for me to use them.' This was another 'not working' issue that Lisa brought to the leadership team. She explained that not all of the staff one-page profiles had enough detailed information about hobbies and interests, which ironically was our first pragmatic reason for introducing them – to match people with staff who shared the same hobby or interest.

We learned that it was very important that the managers had the role of quality checking one-page profiles. This role meant that they took responsibility for the staff one-page profiles being completed and for their quality. The outcome was that we adapted the information sheet about one-page profiles to explain in more detail the importance of having at least two or three specific hobbies and interests on staff one-page profiles.

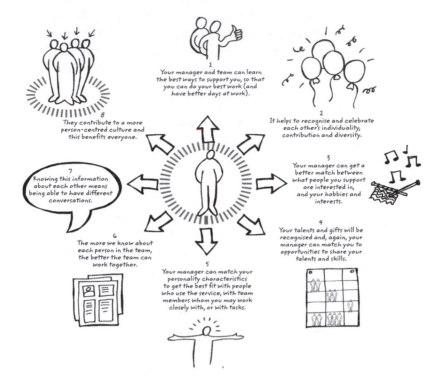

Figure 3.2 The benefits of staff having a one-page profile.

Sharing one-page profiles

When we reviewed our first phase of work with staff in December, one of the administrative staff suggested that the staff one-page profiles were displayed in a staff area, so that all staff could see them. Could we go further than that and have a display of some of the information from staff one-page profiles for families and people living at Bruce Lodge to see? There is a hospital in Blackpool where the nurses and therapists have edited versions of their one-page profiles on the ward for people to read, and this has been a big hit with families and patients. This was an opportunity to share personal information – staff to staff, and with people living at Bruce Lodge and their families.

If you come into Bruce Lodge now, you will see a framed canvas 'Wordle' in the entrance. This is a display of what everyone appreciates about each other – people who live there and staff as well – taken from their one-page profiles. There is also a 'meet the team' book, with all of the staff one-page profiles in it.

Extending to include 'If I could, I would'

As we have explained, the primary purpose of the staff one-page profiles was to be able to match the way that the person living at Bruce Lodge wanted to spend their individual time with a staff member who shared that same hobby or interest.

Could we go further? At the information meetings that started work on each individual's one-page profile, part of the conversation was around 'If I could, I would'. We talked about what else people might want to try or explore, and used this to make decisions about how the person wanted to use their individual time. Joan suggested that it might also be useful for staff to share things that they'd like to do in the future, so that we were not only matchnig people to what staff were doing now in their existing hobbies and interests. It may be that somebody who lived at Bruce Lodge and a staff member both shared something they'd like to do in the future, even though neither of them had direct experience of doing it.

We created a second page, to go after the one-page profile, to ask staff for three opportunities they would like to have. It had an explanation – we were not looking to learn that someone had always wanted to scuba dive off the Great Barrier Reef, but explained how this information would be used in matching them to an individual at Bruce Lodge.

Chapter summary: A one-page profile for every member of staff

We decided to start our project by creating one-page profiles for everyone working at Bruce Lodge for two good reasons. First, the staff at Bruce Lodge would be the key to making our project work so they needed to understand that a person-centred approach included them and how they need to be supported to do great work: the person-centred approach was for them as well as the people living at Bruce Lodge. Second, we needed to know about the staff's interests and hobbies so that we could match them with people who shared them.

In the process of preparing the staff one-page profiles we learned that we needed to explain clearly how the profiles would be used, and to make it easy for staff and their managers to complete their profiles quickly and to a high quality.

In the next chapter we look at how we found out what people living at Bruce Lodge wanted to do with their individual time, how we matched staff with them and how we recorded what they did together.

4

Individual Time

KEN

Ken had been a professional footballer with Stockport County, a fun-loving man with dementia who, for the past three years, has lived at Bruce Lodge. Ken's family sat down with him and some of the team members who knew him best to discuss what they could do to help him, as he appeared to have lost his zest for life and fun. They had several conversations together and developed a one-page profile with Ken. What emerged as really important to Ken were things such as 'sharing his Stockport County memorabilia and old photos', 'watching football on TV' and 'having people around him to enjoy banter with'. Ken will always seek people out and be 'amongst it', as he says.

Lisa looked for someone to match with Ken who was also interested in football and who Ken really got on with.

She chose Sarah. Sarah had never been to a football match, and had always wanted to go: she had listed 'to go to a football match' on the 'If I could, I would' section of her one-page profile. This enabled Ken to be the expert and introduce his passion to Sarah, an opportunity for someone living with dementia to be and feel useful, have a purpose and make a contribution.

Ken says, 'Going to the football again is belting – I felt like I was out there on the pitch again' and 'It's smashing going with Sarah.'

What is important to Ken

- Seeing other people happy!
- Talking about his late wife Doreen.
- Ken and Lynne – his niece and nephew, who visit often.
- The staff team at Bruce Lodge mean the world to Ken and he is to them.
- Loves dancing and a pint of bitter – partying, singing, entertaining.
- Ken bakes, plays dominoes, does crafts – he takes great pleasure from the camaraderie and conversation more than anything!
- "Being in the company of the ladies" – Ken beams when described as a real 'pin up'.
- Having people around him to have banter with. Ken will always seek people out and be 'amongst it', as he says.
- His friendship with Grace.
- Watching football on the TV.
- Showing people his scars from playing football – especially on his leg where he broke it.
- Visiting Stockport County FC for which he used to play, going to the prestigious events at County – as a former player he is always invited and very proud of it.
- Going to watch Stockport County play.
- Sharing his Stockport County memorabilia and old photos, especially the album from his "This is your life" night.
- Having a real man-to-man talk with male staff and visitors
- People watching.
- Chatting about his trade as a painter and decorator.
- Getting out and about – garden centres or a pub lunch are favourite – the busier the better. Ken loves being around people or where there is lots going on.
- Ken loves his bed and 'isn't one for staying up late'.
- 'You can't beat a cooked breakfast' he says.
- Plenty of cups of tea – milk and 2 sugars.
- Biscuits, puddings and treats are a must – due to Ken's recent diagnosis with diabetes these must be monitored – check with a senior. Sunday dinner is favourite.
- Chatting about his retirement on the South Coast – Paignton, Torquay and Dawlish and his love of golf.

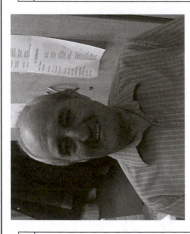

Ken

What those who know Ken best say they like and admire about him

His beaming smile – he lights up the room!

The biggest charmer going!

Sense of fun

"He's so loved"

Always at the heart of things

A real ladies man

Salt of the earth kind of bloke

You just fall in love with Ken!

How we can best support Ken

- Know that Ken gets up in his own time, usually around 8.30 am.
- Be aware that Ken has diabetes – speak to a senior.
- When baking with Ken look for recipes suitable for diabetics.
- Ken is always keen to get to bed but encourage him to have some supper before he goes, so that he isn't hungry. He is usually happy to stay up until 8.30 pm, but if he insists on going earlier, then of course he would go.
- Ken will struggle with lots of stairs or long walks – bear this in mind when arranging to go out with Ken and take a wheelchair if walking any distance or stairs are involved.
- Ken will tell you "his legs have gone" and he may struggle now and again when getting in or out of a chair.
- Ken will use a wheelchair if he gets tired at any time – you will notice he will begin to lean forward.
- Be aware that if Ken goes to County he sits near the touchline to watch the game, and he used to go in the Directors box but that is too high up for him now.
- Ensure Ken has plenty of cups of tea between mealtimes – he will usually have several at breakfast!
- Know that Ken will believe Grace (who lives here) is his late wife Doreen sometimes – respect their friendship, Ken and Grace are fond of each other. Grace is married and as their relationship develops, it is a situation we need to think about together.

Figure 4.1 Ken's one-page profile

Borough *Care*   **Sarah Newcombe**

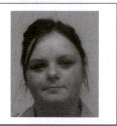

What people like & admire about me
- Hard Working
- Loyal
- Very Friendly
- Lovely to get on with
- Considerate
- Caring

What's important to me...
- My partner Ste and our four children Ellie, Holly, Katie and Ruby, I am a home bird, I love family life.
- Having some time to myself
- Arts and crafts when I can - about once a month
- Visiting Dawlish. I lived there for a few years and my mother-in-law still lives there.
- Reading non-fiction books about anything - a few pages every night
- I enjoy going to the park with my girls at the weekends
- My home and keeping it clean and tidy
- Watching TV, especially Dr Who and Big Brother
- A trip to the cinema about once a month
- That people we support have the best possible lives
- Having time to talk with people living here
- Having fun and banter with my colleagues and people living here

How best to support me...
- If you want me to do a job, just ask, keep things organised – this works best for me.
- If I do anything wrong just tell me, I won't be offended.
- Breaks so that I can phone home and check that everything is OK and have a cigarette.
- I do not find it easy to ask for help, if I am rushing around with lots to do, offer to help.
- Working in bad atmospheres would be a real struggle for me, so to always be open with each other is essential.
- That we all pull together, respect each other and always put the people living here first.

If I could, I would like to try...
1) To go to a football match
2) Arts and crafts, especially painting and drawing
3) Go out for a meal/pub lunches/cafes

The above should be things that you could try together with one of the people living at Bruce Lodge. For example these could be new hobbies or interests that could be shared such as knitting or attending a football match.

Figure 4.2 Sarah's one-page profile

What really matters to you?

Now the staff had one-page profiles, we could start to work with people who lived at Bruce Lodge to find out how they wanted to use their individual time. We began to have informal meetings with individuals, their families and staff to learn more about what really mattered to each person, how they wanted to be supported and how they wanted to use their individual time. We did this by arranging an hour-and-a-half meeting with the individual, their family, Lisa and ideally another staff member. These were simply called 'one-page profile meetings'. Gill initially facilitated each meeting.

Calling them 'meetings' may give the wrong impression. They were purposeful conversations. Gill began by talking about what a good day and a bad day looked like for this person, as a way both to learn what was important to them, and what good support looked like. She also asked what it would take to create more good days for them.

We've given examples of what people told us in these meetings below.

People's good and bad days

- A good day for Winifred used to be spent tidying and cleaning the house. This was clearly very important to Winifred, and her daughters described her as a wonderful homemaker.

- Helen told us that a good day for her was seeing Lynn, her daughter, and going to the hairdresser's.

- For Ken a bad day would be if people around him were miserable, and he was spending a lot of time alone, bored, and a good day is when he watches football, and has a cooked breakfast.

- Ellen was very clear that 'good' for her meant watching the squirrels playing in the garden and feeding the birds.

What was working and not working

Gill would introduce questions around what was working and not working for the person, from the family's perspective, and Lisa would contribute her own perspective as well.

- Winifred could not directly say what was working and not working for her, but her daughters, Maureen and Bernie, said that their best guess was that what was working was seeing her family, her grandchildren and great grandchildren, and what was not working was when people leave, as this distresses her, and people wanting her to get dressed and go to bed when she was not in the mood.

- Lisa thought that what was working for Helen was when her room was homely and she was surrounded by her favourite things, and what was not working was that Helen loves animals and does not have many opportunities to see or be with them.

- Ken said that what was working for him was his family visiting and staff having a laugh and joke with him, and what was not working for him was not seeing enough football.

If I could, I would: How I want to use my time

Gill also asked about 'If I could, I would', and specifically how the person would like to use their two hours.

- Ken wanted see Stockport County play.

- Marie clearly said that she wanted to go back to her church and attend Mass.

- Ellen wanted to visit the war memorial for animals lost in the war.

- Helen wanted to go walking with a dog and be in touch with her daughter when she is in Dubai.

- Winifred's family and Lisa decided together that what would make her happiest was to be involved in the household chores within the home.

These structured conversations gave Gill enough information to pull together a one-page profile for each person and to have a really clear picture of how they wanted to use their two hours.

Gathering information from everyone

Of course, some people who live at Bruce Lodge don't use words to speak, but it was still really important that they were at the meetings. Staff, and most importantly families, shared their knowledge and insights to help make best guesses together about what was important to the person, what good support looked like from their perspective and how they might want to use their time.

Matching staff to what the person wanted to do

With the information we gathered from the people living at Bruce Lodge and the staff one-page profiles, Lisa was able to suggest a good match between what the person wanted to do and a staff member. She did this by looking at existing good relationships, and most importantly for an activity that a staff member was either already doing or wanted to do that matched the activity that the individual had identified. This process would usually give Lisa a couple of staff members who she could suggest to the person for them to choose from, though sometimes there was only one person who shared the interest for Lisa to suggest.

We deliberately did not simply use the person's existing key worker to deliver the activity they had chosen. We wanted to get the best match from across the staff team, and this included staff who were non-contact staff, such as housekeepers and administrators.

We also learned from the individual and their family about when in the day the person would ideally want their two hours. They might prefer their two hours in one block, split into one hour every other week, or even into half an hour a week, depending on what the activity was.

A summary of the process
Gather information from the meeting

- Gather information for the one-page profile.

- Outcome for the individual – how do they want to use their time?

- Other information for matching to a staff member (who they get on with now, the characteristics of the people they get on with best).

Look at staff one-page profiles

- Find the best match based on shared interests (either ones that are important to the staff member now or that they would like to try).

- From the staff who share this interest, find the best match based on existing relationships and the kind of person the individual gets on with. The appreciation section from the staff one-page profiles helped with this as well.

- Share the options with the person for them to choose if there is more than one possibility.

Putting the process into practice

Lisa's challenge was to put all this on the rota and make sure that it happened! Lisa said:

I got to know the staff profiles very well as I had to keep looking at them to do the matching! Sometimes there were several possible people; sometimes, like with Marie and Olivia, there was only one obvious match. I would talk to the person about possible matches to see who their preference was, but some people just wanted me to decide. It was a completely different way to do the rota. Now I had to do it around when people wanted to have their individual time. That was a challenge at first.

We started small and slowly, with just three meetings in May, arranging the individual hours with three people. As Lisa's confidence and experience grew, more and more meetings took place. The rota became increasingly challenging to develop, but Lisa managed it. By October everybody had had a meeting, everybody had their outcomes in place, and they were starting to experience their individual time.

We asked staff to take a photograph during each session of individual time, and complete a learning log straight afterwards.

Learning logs

Every service requires a record of what happened during the day, and staff at Bruce Lodge used daily records. As individual time was new, we wanted to make sure that we reflected and learned from how it went. This could tell us more about the person and how to support them well. Learning logs were the ideal tool for this.

After four or five learning logs have been filled in about a person, the senior looks at the information they contain and uses it to update the person's one-page profile. The learning log is likely to reveal new information about both what is important to the person, and how best to support them (and possibly appreciations too).

Unlike traditional progress notes, learning logs can inform changes to both the one-page profile and how the person spends their time, because we can pull out things that have worked really well that may reflect additional information about what's important to somebody. They also say what's not worked so well that needs to be different next time, which can help us in further informing how best to support the person.

For example, to ensure that Winifred continues to be supported in a way that makes sense to her, Beryl completes a learning log whenever she works with her.

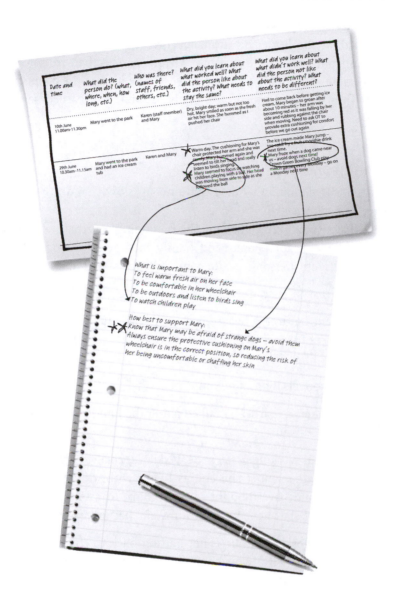

Figure 4.3 Using information from a learning log to update the one-page profile

What worked and what didn't work

As usual, at the leadership team meeting we looked at what was working and not working from a staff perspective, from Gill's perspective and from Lisa's perspective. By looking at the comments cards from families and professionals as well, we learned several things.

What worked

Lisa said 'It definitely worked building up slowly, and just trying three this month.'

What also worked right from the beginning was that staff could see the benefits for people, and family members responded very positively. Here are some of the comments from staff about this:

'It is great to see the satisfaction on people's faces.'

'Jan went out to the beauty parlour to have her nails done, and then went for a glass of wine with the staff supporting her and had a ball!'

'Good conversations are going on.'

Family members in particular talked about the importance of people being matched well.

'I think it is working great, she loved it, especially being matched with a staff member she enjoys being with, doing things we never would have thought – even going to a bike show. The member of staff matched to Mum visits her in hospital too.'

'What is working for me is her getting back to church, and the fact that my wife is matched with a staff member who likes going to church too.'

What didn't work

LEARNING ABOUT LEARNING LOGS

'The learning logs are not always being filled in, or with enough detail', Gill found.

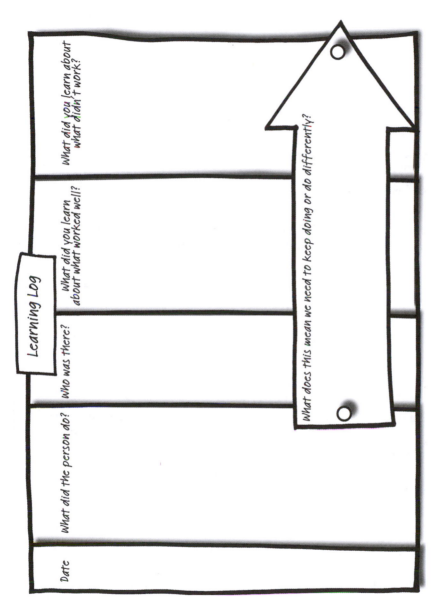

Figure 4.4 Learning log

Lisa agreed that this was not happening consistently and that the quality of the information was variable. We recognised that it would have been helpful to include learning logs in the initial training that staff had done (the half a day on one-page profiles). Our action was to develop several best practice examples, and a summary of what a learning log is and how it is used, in the same way as we had done for the one-page profile. Gill and Lisa then invested more time in coaching and supporting staff to complete them. Soon they were being done to a high standard and taking no more than ten minutes.

PHOTOS: MAKING SURE THEY HAPPEN AND ARE SHARED

'We are not getting many photos – staff forget to take the camera', said Kerri.

It was a challenge for staff to remember to take a photo every time people went out to create a record of the activity. We tried different ways to remind people to take photos. The one that we ended up with is that if you go to Bruce Lodge now, there'll be a sticker on the door as you leave saying 'If you're going out on individual time, we hope you remember the camera.' We needed to provide two cameras to make that happen, and explored different ways of getting the photos printed out and made available to people in their folders.

SHARING INFORMATION WITH FAMILIES

On one of the comment cards, a family member made an important point that made us think about how the photos were being shared, and how we kept families informed. The daughter said 'Mum could not tell me that she had been swimming, so I could not talk to her about it. It would have been good to have known in advance if possible.' We recognised that we needed to use the photos and learning logs better to make sure family members knew when individual time was happening, and could see how well it had gone.

Now Lisa phones family members the week before the individual time is going to happen to tell them about it. And we make sure the photo and the learning log are available in the file in the individual's room for family members to see, so they can have a conversation with the person about their activity.

Chapter summary: Sarah and Ken went to football, and Winifred cleaned and tidied

Now we could really get going. Starting slowly at first, we began to find out about people's interests, to match them with staff who shared the same interest, and they began to use their individual time.

Matching people and designing a rota around individual time was complicated at first, but the effect on the people living at Bruce Lodge was wonderful to see.

We recorded people's individual time by using learning logs, and these helped us to improve people's profiles so we could give them better support in the future.

In the next chapter we look at how the culture changed at Bruce Lodge, and what this meant for the way everyone worked.

5

Four Plus
One Questions

WINIFRED

Winifred is described as a wonderfully loving personality who brightens the room with her smile (see Figure 5.1). Winifred's daughters and the team recognised that Winifred was feeling lost at times. The greatest struggle for Winifred's two daughters Maureen and Bernie was saying goodbye to her after they'd visited. Often Winifred could be seen at the locked gate of the home, crying on her knees and searching for her daughters.

Lisa and Gill spent an hour with Winifred, Maureen and Bernie to develop her one-page profile. They focused on what made good days and bad days for Winifred, past and present. They talked about what was going well and what needed to change. Winifred's daughters described her as a wonderful homemaker, and said that for her a good day would be spent tidying and cleaning the house: this was clearly very important to Winifred. They decided together that what would make Winifred happiest was to be involved in the household chores within the home. The next decision was who she wanted to support her.

It only took a little lateral thinking to realise that Beryl, the housekeeper, was the natural choice to support Winifred. Winifred and Beryl got along well together, so it felt as though it was a real win–win situation. They shared an interest in looking after the cleaning and the domestic chores, as well as having a really good relationship.

Winifred's new relationship with Beryl and extra responsibility has had an extraordinary effect on her happiness and well-being. At home she would routinely clean the house, so before this was identified in the one-page profile as being important to her, a big part of her life and identity had been missing.

Maureen and Bernie, Winifred's daughters, have noticed the change that the one-page profile and individual time has made to Winifred. She is happier, chatting more, using fuller sentences, sleeping better and is generally more alive. Maureen says:

The difference is astounding: Mum was a housewife, a practical person who spent her life caring for her five children and our father, who died 20 years ago. Her desire to care for people was never blunted but the ability to do so was robbed from her and that left her very frustrated. These chores are helping her connect with other things from her past and are opening up new pathways in her mind. The first thing that we noticed had come back was her language – within a week of working with Beryl she was recalling words much better and introducing me to other people by name, whereas before she didn't know who I was.

Winifred now has more choice and control over how she lives her life and how she is supported on a day-to-day basis. The staff have created an environment that says 'We've plenty of jobs for you to do.' Winifred can often be seen late in the evening folding laundry that the staff have left, or hanging the wet washing over the maiden. Nothing makes Winifred happier than being outside on a fine breezy day and hanging the washing out on the washing line.

Another positive spin-off that Maureen talks about is that Winifred's genuine kindness to other people has returned as a result of this new role she's taken within the home. It seems to have brought back her mum's unusual sensitivity and empathy to anyone in sight. Maureen shared an observation she'd made when she sat in the lounge with Winifred. Another lady in the lounge was confused and seemed to be increasingly upset. Winifred left her chair in mid-sentence and walked away from Maureen. She slowly approached this lady and bent down to her level, saying 'I can see you're upset about something. Look, I'm stroking your hand to make you feel better. I'm Winifred, and you can talk to me anytime, love.' The lady cried and Winifred wiped her tears away. Winifred cried and she wiped her own tears away. Then they smiled at each other as though joined in a private sisterhood. Maureen says her heart was filled with emotion, and pride for Winifred.

Winifred is delightfully mischievous, and Maureen says her personality has really come to life again. Winifred's story is a great example of the huge difference this approach can make to people.

What is important to Winifred

- Her daughters Bernie and Maureen who visit daily.

- Pat her daughter who travels up from London to visit and Marie who lives in Liverpool and visits fortnightly.

- Seeing Kevin and David, who are Bernie and Maureen's spouses – they remind Winifred of her brothers.

- Her grandchildren, Terence, Emma and Ria. Also her great grandchildren, Grace, Ben, Harry, Zach, Charlie, Jack and Oliver. Winifred has a new great grandchild due later on in the year (June 2012).

- Not to be around people who swear or are vulgar.

- Winifred visibly grows when complimented – do this often!

- Her Roman Catholic faith. Winifred must say her prayers each morning and evening.

- She adores cups of tea – milk no sugar.

- Her rapport with Beryl. Winifred loves to be involved in household chores – folding the home's laundry is a must and she loves to clean.

- Kisses and cuddles – Winifred is very tactile and loves a hug. A big smile will draw her to you.

- A diet which works for her – good quality food has always been important to Winifred. She always loved Marks and Spencer's food, fish, salmon, vegetables and a light breakfast.

- Company is vital to Winifred – spending time with others, especially Grace, Doreen, John and Joan, who live with Winifred.

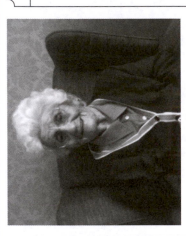

Winifred

What those who know Winifred best say they like and admire about her

A wonderfully loving personality.

She brightens the room with her smile.

Her warmth.

Her beautiful nature and generosity of spirit.

She restores my faith in human nature.

How we can best support Winifred

- Be aware that Winifred is afraid of water – she does not/must not shower or bathe but thoroughly strip washes herself each day with a supporter nearby.

- Know that Winifred is often preoccupied in the morning. She must sort her room out before she does anything. Give her time and space to do this. She will appreciate you taking her a cup of tea whilst she does this.

- Know that Winifred will worry about upsetting her tummy and the need to let things settle after eating, always respect what she is telling you around this and go with her on it.

- Winifred will eat a light breakfast mid morning and loves to sit and chat as she eats.

- If Winifred is reluctant to get ready for bed, to avoid her becoming distressed, divert her by talking about saying her prayers together with you – ask Winifred to start you off as you have forgotten the prayer.

- Know that Winifred is not a lover of TV and should be supported in 'doing'. She will become bored and fractious if left sitting for long periods.

Figure 5.1 Winifred's one-page profile

Personalisation: Embedding cultural change

Our monthly leadership meetings – and the structure that we put in to learn what was working and not working – gave us lots of opportunities to think about what else we needed do to really embed the cultural and practical changes that personalisation required. In this chapter we share four of the questions that we needed to answer, and the changes that this process required for the way that staff and managers worked.

What if…the person changes their mind?
…or the staff member is off sick?

This was one of the challenges that Lisa raised at one of the leadership team meetings. What happened if when we got to the time when the person was supposed to be doing their activities, either the staff member was off sick or the individual no longer wanted to do the activity? We used one of our leadership team meetings to think this through and create a detailed flowchart to look at the different possibilities.

An analogy is going to the hairdresser's. Most people have their favourite stylist and would make an appointment to have their hair cut with them. Let's imagine you have an appointment to have your hair cut with Lesley on Saturday. If on Saturday you suddenly have an opportunity to meet up with an old friend who is unexpectedly in the area, and choose to cancel your hair appointment, you would need to wait until Lesley could fit you in again. If you arrived for your appointment and Lesley was off sick, the hairdresser's would be responsible for finding someone else to do your hair. If you only wanted Lesley, then you could rearrange for when Lesley was back.

We decided that if a staff member was sick, it was still our responsibility to provide the individual time then and to offer another person to support the individual time. The person could choose whether to continue or wait for their 'Lesley' to be back. If the person changed their mind about the activity, and no longer wanted to do it that day, we would then rearrange it for them. If they changed their mind about what they wanted to do (e.g. it was raining and they no longer wanted to go out), we would offer them a Plan B (something that they wanted to do that did not involve going out).

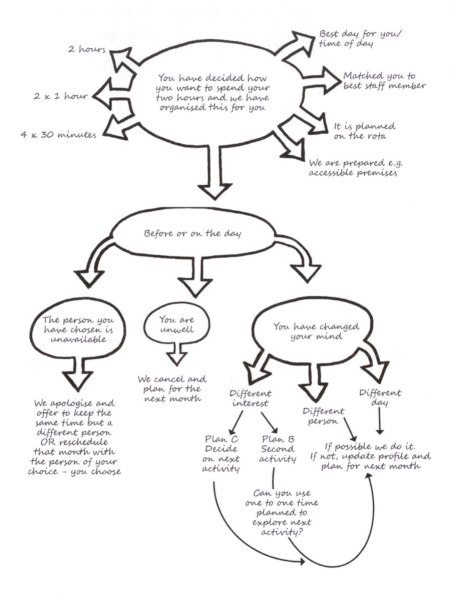

Figure 5.2 What if?

This really helped us understand that we needed to have a backup planned outcome (Plan B) for the individual. On the basis of this, when we continued to do the meetings with individuals to find out how they wanted to use their time, we would talk about a backup plan as well.

How can we pay for staff expenses?

Another challenge that was raised – again by both family members and staff – was around who should pay for staff to have teas and coffees, or entrance to the swimming baths, for example. We decided that it wasn't appropriate to ask the individual themselves to fund this.

Each home in Borough Care had an activities budget that typically got used in a broader activities programme. Ines and Lisa agreed that they would deconstruct that activities budget and individualise it for each person (i.e. divide it between 43 people). This would provide the money to support staff to go out in their personalisation time. We called it the personalisation support budget instead of the activities budget. This meant that staff were enabled to go and support individuals to do the outcome they wanted, particularly in the community.

This put pressure on the home to raise more money to cover the deficit for the activities budget to make sure that things like the Christmas party and the summer fair were still able to happen.

How can we make sure we are not duplicating paperwork?

This was a concern raised by Ines, the deputy CEO, about the impact of what we were doing on the paperwork at Bruce Lodge. In fact, the one-page profiles became the first page of the care files held about individuals. Learning logs were used to update the one-page profiles, and this made sure that they stayed up to date and reflected any changes that were happening for the person as their dementia progressed.

In the first three or four months Lisa took responsibility for looking at the learning logs and using these to update the one-page profiles. After that, she supported the seniors to do this. They arranged to have an extended handover to look at the learning logs with the staff member who was doing the individual time.

How can we be more creative in supporting people to use their individual time?

We spent an hour in a leadership team meeting helping Lisa and Gill to think about creative ways that people could use their individual time to achieve their outcome. We asked Lisa to bring eight examples of individual outcomes that people wanted to achieve. For each one, we thought about:

- If you were going to do this in the community – where would you go?

- If you wanted to meet others who shared this interest – where would you go?

- If you were going to do this in Bruce Lodge – how could you do this?

- What could we do for free?

- What could we do if there was some funding?

Here is an example:

Table 5.1 Example of creative support for individual time

John was interested in using his two hours around gardening.	
If I were going to do this in the community – where would I go?	Garden centre
If I wanted to meet others who shared this interest – where would I go?	At the garden centre there are weekly sessions for gardeners to join, with coffee afterwards. Is there a local allotment society? There is a local group looking at sustainable living and this includes creating urban herb gardens – could John join this? Match with a volunteer who has a garden and help them in the garden.
If I were going to do this in Bruce Lodge – how could I do this?	Talk to the cooks about John growing herbs either indoors or outdoors.
What could I do for free?	Have a seed/plant collection – ask staff and visitors to help us create a herb garden or plant area in one of the planters in the courtyard area.
What could I do if there was some funding?	Look at a garden area with a potting bench and shed.

This is one example of how personalisation meant thinking differently. Most care homes have a garden area where people can sit. Actually getting involved in gardening, particularly without extra funding, requires flexible thinking, but the team proved to be extremely creative once they saw the possibilities available and the difference the activity might make to someone.

This is the key to the cultural change that everyone at Bruce Lodge experienced: their involvement in creating one-page profiles and individual time really did mean that they began truly to see the people they worked with as individuals.

What this means for the way staff work

Personalisation requires a cultural change from a task-focused ethos to one that values what matters most to the people being supported. We needed to work with staff to help them think about the language they used, being prepared and routines.

Language

When we started this project, we heard people being described with words like 'feeders', 'doubles' and 'singles', which referred to whether people needed support at meal times and whether they needed help from one or two people with personal care. Lisa needed to work with her staff on the power of language, what language was acceptable and to be encouraged, and what language we didn't want to use at Bruce Lodge. At the leadership team meeting we looked at what support we could give Lisa.

The term 'residents' was commonly used at Bruce Lodge, in the leadership team as well as among staff. So we stopped talking about people as 'residents', and talked about people as being individuals who lived at Bruce Lodge.

Being prepared

Another example of how staff needed to work differently was being prepared for the individual time. On one occasion a taxi had to wait for 15 minutes because the staff member who was supporting the individual with their time didn't have everything arranged.

Lisa had to work with staff and seniors to make sure that people saw themselves as responsible for being completely ready before the individual time started, rather than using some of the time to make sure people had everything they needed.

Being flexible

One of the concerns that staff raised when talking about what wasn't working was 'people taking their individual time out at times when we're busy', such as near lunchtimes. Lisa did everything she could to try to make sure that people weren't having their individual time around lunchtime, but of course that was sometimes unavoidable (for example, going to church meant that people were coming back around lunchtime). This was an example of starting to move from a task culture to one that focused more on relationships.

What this means for managers

To continue to build the cultural change that was emerging meant that we needed to support Lisa and the seniors to give people great feedback about what they were doing well, and to feed back quickly and appropriately about things that needed to change.

Gill and Lisa looked together at how to structure the supervision sessions that seniors have with staff, and that Lisa was having with seniors. They considered different ways of coaching and feedback, and how to make sure they were effective.

Catching people doing something well, and giving them good feedback on this, is not typically characteristic of care home management. For Lisa, Kerri and the seniors, supporting staff as described in their one-page profiles, giving them feedback and coaching them in using person-centred practices (for example learning logs) was a new way of working.

What else did we learn?

As well as solving problems, and refining the practicalities of implementing personalisation, as a leadership team we were also learning about the change process. We learnt that we had been overambitious in one area and that we needed to keep working on getting feedback from families.

We were overambitious

Our dashboard told us that we weren't doing as well on communication charts and decision-making agreements as we'd hoped. When we first started we'd hoped that every individual would have both a communication chart and a decision-making agreement. We quickly learned that this was just too much to achieve in the first phase of this work.

So we decided together that we would have communication charts or decision-making agreements when for whatever reason they seemed particularly important for an individual. We used them, for example, when someone didn't use words to speak at all, or if we had particular concerns about decision-making. But we decided that we'd really look at developing communication charts and decision-making agreements further in Phase 2 of the work that we were doing together.

Working at getting continuous feedback from families

Another thing we noticed was that after the first couple of months we weren't getting as many feedback cards from relatives. We decided to be much more proactive about this: we gave relatives the feedback card in the first planning meeting that we did with people to develop the one-page profile, and encouraged them to return them. This made a big difference to the number of feedback comments cards that we received.

Chapter summary: Solving problems and embracing change

This is a project that's designed to radically improve people's lives. It's based on changing the way we think about people who live in care homes, so that we listen to what they want and find ways of bringing it about by giving them time, opportunity and real choices.

The process of doing this is bound to cause some practical difficulties, and to challenge the way some people think about their work. As a team we tackled the challenges, found solutions and worked hard at helping everyone to embrace the new way of working that the project brought into the home.

In the next chapter, we look at how we analysed our progress so far, and made plans for the next stage.

6

What Next?

ELAINE

Elaine was becoming more and more unwell, and it became clearer that she was moving towards the end of her life. Gill, Elaine's family and the staff who more closely supported Elaine completed 'Living well, and planning for the end of your life' with Elaine. This is a fill-in booklet that uses person-centred practices to help people think about their end-of-life wishes. This ensured they were having conversations before Elaine was too poorly to tell them her wishes, or her family too distressed to focus their attention.

Lisa and the staff did some additional assessments to work out how to make sure Elaine was as comfortable as possible and they reviewed her pain control. They did noise assessments (and visual, tactile and multiple stress assessments) to consider Elaine's environment and they developed an action plan to reduce the noise levels around her room, where she was spending more and more of her time. Elaine's one-page profile was updated to reflect the changes in her life and health.

Here is some of what was important to Elaine at that time:

- Seeing Sandra and Rose, her two daughters, each week – they must bring fresh flowers!

- Sitting in the quieter areas with someone to sit by her and lead a conversation

- Sitting where she could see what was going on in and around the home: Elaine loves to look out of the window at what is happening outdoors

- Not being in the dark

- Being with babies and children

- Listening to music some time each day – Daniel O'Donnell is Elaine's favourite

- Her Roman Catholic faith: Elaine would pray often; seeing Father Bulfin, the local priest, who called monthly

- A warm bath three or four times a week.

Here is a snippet of what you would have needed to know if you were responsible for supporting Elaine:

- Always support Elaine to sit where she can look out of the window – chat with her about the birds in the garden and when it is warm help her into the garden to feed the birds.

- Always make sure that there is a light on in her room, as the dark frightens Elaine.

- Find any opportunity for Elaine to cuddle a baby or watch small children play.

As Elaine's dementia and physical condition deteriorated over the following six months:

- She would now 'grab' at staff as they came close.

- She was totally dependent on others for eating, drinking, moving and all personal care.

- She would sit picking at the chair, her skin, materials – retreating within her inner self.

- She no longer used words to speak.

The staff made changes to Elaine's environment to reflect both what was important to her and the support she needed. Her bed was placed by the window, and given her love of birds, a bird table was put in her view. Her room always had at least one vase of fresh flowers; her bed was regularly moved to give differing views. Staff looked at how to reduce the reflective tiling and glare in Elaine's room. Tactile assessments and multiple stress assessments had also been carried out and acted on. Staff were far more alert to ensuring sheets were wrinkle free, and used the gentlest touch – small but vital points that made a difference to Elaine and were recorded on her one-page profile.

Staff and Elaine's daughters began to recite her favourite prayers to her each evening. Elaine would stroke your hand on occasions when looking directly into your eyes. Elaine seemed to get the greatest comfort from having a bath, so this was planned several times a week. Her bathroom, which had previously been sterile and clinical, was now a warm, inviting place for her to have a relaxing bath in – very soft fluffy towels were a must! Daniel O'Donnell music would play gently as she soaked, and beautifully coloured throws covered the necessary equipment when it wasn't in use.

Lisa and Elaine's family decided to change her two hours' individual time to five-minute sessions every hour, where the member of staff chosen to work with Elaine would sit and connect with her, and simply be with her. Without focused effort we knew this would not happen and so Elaine's individual time was structured very differently at this point. The staff who had now been matched to work with Elaine, and Elaine's daughters, also explored ideas from the information we had gathered earlier, to increase the quality and quantity of connections with Elaine. They came up with a whole list of ideas from massage and audiobooks to placing meaningful pictures in her view. Staff brought their babies and pets in to see Elaine, she was given freshly laundered baby clothes to smell, staff would sit alongside Elaine on the bed and hold her whilst looking through her cherished photo albums – we observed a calm and relaxed Elaine during many of these attempts to truly connect with her.

Staff assumed that Elaine understood at some level any comments made in her presence, and every task was now seen as an opportunity to talk, and through gentle touch, to connect with Elaine.

Elaine passed away peacefully during the night. Her daughter Rose said how much the care her mum received during the last months of her life meant to her: 'I don't know how they did it with 40-odd people here, but it felt like it was only my mum being looked after. She was looked after so well, right to the end.'

Taking stock and planning the next phase

By the end of October everybody living at Bruce Lodge had a one-page profile, and everybody was using their individual time. Phase 1 was complete. The leadership team decided to take stock and do a more detailed analysis of what was working and what was not working so that we could continue to improve, and plan a second phase of our work to start in January.

In our first phase – described in Chapters 1 to 5 – the leadership team decided what we were going to try to achieve and how we were going to do this. In Phase 2, we wanted the staff to be much more directly involved in determining what we wanted to do as we took the project wider and deeper.

Listening to staff

It was not possible to get the entire staff team together and off rota – so we went to them. Instead of the December leadership team meeting, three of us visited Bruce Lodge to meet as many staff as possible, to find out what staff thought and what they wanted to see happen next.

Two of us camped out in the office, and another member of the leadership team spent time with people and staff in the communal rooms, having individual conversations about how it was going. We put a pinboard up in the office, with four columns – the name of the staff member, what they thought was going well/working, what they thought was not working/could be improved, and what they would like to see happen next. Whenever a staff member popped into the office we would ask them if we could have ten minutes, ask them the questions and write their answers on the board. One of the catering assistants, Catherine, came in first, looking for Lisa to sign off an order. She looked a bit shocked to be asked her opinion (and for her name to go up first).

Catherine said that not all staff were able to look at each other's one-page profiles. For example, as a member of the kitchen staff she wasn't always able to see what was on the one-page profiles of the other staff. She asked, 'Could we have them somewhere where all staff could see them?' in the next phase.

What was working?

Here are some of the things that staff said were working:
Kerri said:

> It was lovely to hear stories from people themselves and from staff. It was absolutely brilliant that people were doing these things, something of their choice in their one-to-one time. And their families are really intrigued. Many of them know what we're doing, and there are lots and lots of enquiries about vacancies; in fact, they have doubled in the last two months. And three-quarters of the people who are phoning up about enquiries are specifically mentioning the one-to-one or personalisation time.

Kerri added that it is 'nice to see people going out to different places, and the getting ready and the excitement of going places'. She thought that 'people were really opening up and their personalities showing through the one-to-one.'

Margaret said how exciting it was to hear success stories like Winifred's, and she noticed that 'people were having better relationships with staff and were remembering staff's names because of the one-to-one sessions they were doing together.' She talked about a couple of people like Bessie who had been noticeably calmer, and thought that one-to-one time with Bessie had really helped her.

Similarly, Joy talked about a couple of the success stories from her perspective and said one of the great things for her was going swimming with May.

Beryl talked about the person she was matched with, Winifred. Beryl saw Winifred's personality coming out and that she was becoming more of the person that she once was, and Beryl saw Winifred's sense of humour again. Beryl mentioned developing the relationships between individuals and staff and how important that had been. She said there was nothing that she wanted to change. She was happily giving her time to be matched to an individual and didn't feel out of her depth at all, which was something that people were concerned about as she was not a member of care staff.

Maz said 'how brilliant it was finding out more about people's interests and what was important to them. And seeing the difference it made to people spending time with people doing the things that they want to do.'

Karen also talked about how spending time with people was 'building and developing relationships between staff and individuals who lived there.'

Marion talked about how much she was enjoying doing something the person wished to do, and the good job getting a good match had been.

We describe what staff said was not working, and their other suggestions for the future, later in this chapter, as part of our 'four plus one questions'.

We managed to get over a third of the staff team to contribute their views over the two hours. We left the pinboard up, and Lisa and Kerri supported staff over the next three weeks to add their perspectives as well.

We used the feedback from staff to contribute to a bigger review and reflection that took place at our leadership team meeting in January. We used the reflections from staff, and more comment cards from relatives and professionals to do a 'four plus one' analysis.

Four plus one questions

'Four plus one' is another person-centred thinking tool that is powerful for reflecting on progress and learning, and using this to inform next steps. The following summaries integrate the feedback from staff, families and the leadership team.

The first question: What had we tried?

The first question is simply a way to document what we have tried. We went back to the one-page strategy to help inform this and created a factual, full list of what we had tried over the ten months since April. Here is our list:

- a one-page strategy and dashboard to track progress

- one-page profiles for everyone who lived at Bruce Lodge

- 'If I could, I would' and 'working and not working' (with actions) for everyone

- training for staff on one-page profiles

- using templates for one-page profiles – staff and individuals

- Gill coaching Lisa, Kerri and the seniors

- staff have one-page profiles and 'If I could, I would'

- matching staff to how people wanted to spend their individual time

- writing the rota around individual time

- staff doing learning logs after individual time

- taking photos of each individual time

- changing the activities budget to a personalisation support budget to cover staff expenses for individual time

- getting comments from relatives and professionals through comments cards

- monthly feedback from staff, managers and Gill through 'working and not working'

- monthly leadership team meetings to problem-solve and keep track of progress

- implementing a communication strategy that included stories, video and social media – Lisa had been interviewed on local radio, and our work had been featured in the local press, *Community Care* and *The Guardian*.

The second question: What have we learned?

- Lisa said that she had learned that people could do new things that you don't usually see happen in care homes – she'd seen an 84-year-old go swimming each month, someone going to a wine bar after they had had their nails done, and another using Skype to stay in touch with family.

- We learned that this was really being driven by Lisa and supported by Kerri, but we hadn't got to the stage where it felt like common practice and just the way things happened around here. We needed to work much harder to get all the seniors on board and to make it just the way we do things.

- Introducing one-page profiles and 'personalisation time' had had a positive effect on the culture, with staff knowing people as individuals, and supporting them as individuals in their day-to-day care and support. Jeannie, a staff member, said that 'spending time with people made such a big difference over what we were doing before of just taking care of people's daily care needs. And what a difference it had made finding out more about people'.

- Staff were very positive about their own hobbies and interests being taken into account, and having their own one-page profiles. Lisa talked about seeing staff going the extra mile in ways she had not seen before. Helen loves dogs, and is matched to Rosalind who has a dog. Rosalind comes in early for her 3 pm shift, and brings her dog with her so that she can walk the dog with Helen. Rosalind then leaves her dog with Helen for the rest of her shift, which is as close as we have been able to get to Helen owning a dog.

When Rosalind is not working, she sometimes comes and collects Helen to walk the dog with her.

- Lisa described how supporting staff to do their one-page profiles and using their interests to match people had made a really big impact on staff morale. She was impressed with the staff's commitment to making it happen. Lisa described it as people being a 'really special group committed to making this happen'.

- We learned that on-site coaching is crucial. Lisa said that Gill's coaching was incredibly significant in supporting her to implement this and to make sure that the meetings took place.

- We also learned that although having information about people's histories had been useful, it was much more important to know what matters to people now and to have the detail about how they wanted to be supported.

- Sharing one-page profiles at handovers had been really important, and using learning logs to ensure that they were updated.

The third question: What were we pleased about?

- We were pleased about the way that Lisa had taken this challenge, and that everyone had individual time within ten months. We were pleased about the difference made by the two hours a month that people now had in their lives, as well as the difference that it had made to their day-to-day support.

- We were pleased that staff were bringing the whole of themselves to work and seeing people beyond their dementia.

- We were pleased at the depth of conversations and honesty that we'd had in the leadership meetings, and that we focused on what was working and what wasn't working. It was really important for us to meet together monthly to stay on track around this and how the different roles and responsibilities within the leadership team had worked. The one-page strategy gave us a clear direction, and the dashboard had been really helpful in making sure we stuck to it. Managers keeping a journal of what was working and not working, and us all having continuous ways for monitoring how we were doing, had been really important as well.

- We were also pleased that the project had made a difference to Borough Care as a whole, as it was now included in their dementia strategy.

- We were pleased that we put a communication strategy in place right from the beginning, and that we had paid attention to recording stories to share.

- We were pleased at how families were really engaged with the process. Lisa gave examples of families bringing in items for other people's individual time, for example books about Stockport County for Ken.

- We were pleased that the project had had an impact on how Bruce Lodge was seen. Enquiries at Bruce Lodge had doubled, and three-quarters of families enquiring specifically mentioned individual time.

The fourth question: What were we concerned about?

- Lisa thought that staff could sometimes give up on people who seemed more set in their ways, so we needed to find different ways of encouraging people to try new things, or to learn about things in different ways.

- Initially people hadn't been so good at completing learning logs, and we've learned that we need to train on learning logs at the same time as one-page profiles.

- The project meant that individuals and families had much higher expectations of the service they were receiving at Bruce Lodge. This meant that people felt more comfortable sharing their niggles as well. While this felt like a good thing overall, obviously if you were the person receiving those niggles (i.e. Lisa) it didn't always feel so positive!

- One of Lisa's concerns was whether, if she or Kerri wasn't there, the process was still happening. Making sure it was firmly part of the culture was something that we worried about. How could we make sure the new way of working went from project to habit? How would we make sure all staff shared equal responsibility for it, particularly the seniors, and it wasn't just seen as something that Lisa was doing?

- How could we make sure that night staff really, really felt involved in this as well?

- Given that we'd changed the activities budget to make it a supporting personalisation budget, how could we make sure there was still enough money to do other things that people wanted to do?

- The new seniors had told us that they were finding it hard to fit things in. Learning about a new job role and a new structure was problematic for some people. In addition, staff weren't always taking photos.

- While two hours a month was much better than people had before, it wasn't possible to use any more paid staff to take things further, so we needed to find more and different ways to get people to have more time.

- One family member said that she was really, really pleased with the individual time. But she asked us to make sure that we weren't failing to attend enough to group activities. And she was right. We'd focused so much on the individual time that there weren't a lot of structured group activities happening as well.

- How could we make more and better connections outside Bruce Lodge with organisations that could help us to deliver individual time as well as the staff?

The 'plus one' question: What were we going to do next?

The staff had made specific suggestions about what they wanted to happen next. Here they are:

- Kerri suggested that we made sure that one-page profiles went out with people, so they were used when people went for hospital and medical appointments (this now happens).

- Margaret wondered whether we could link to volunteer groups to increase the number of hours that people had.

- Another staff member asked 'Could we have different ways for people to capture what they did in their one-to-one time?' For example, creating photo albums for people would be great for families to see, or photographs to keep on digital photo frames so people could keep seeing photos of the things they were doing going around in a loop.

- Kerri also talked about whether there could be more ideas of places to go, and she suggested that the photos be displayed so that everybody could see them.

All the leadership team voted on the staff suggestions, and on key areas arising from the four plus one questions. This enabled us to decide what we wanted to focus on for the last six months of the project. What did we need to do to really embed the changes and build on them?

From the voting we identified nine key goals that we wanted to achieve. They incorporated the staff's suggestions, our concerns and the fact that as a leadership team we wanted to learn what people living at Bruce Lodge wanted to change by using the process called Working Together for Change (described in Chapter 8).

Here are the goals we wanted to focus on:

1. We wanted to have a way for people living at Bruce Lodge to share what they were doing with each other, using photos and other means.

2. It was really important that we went from this being a project to it being a habit. We needed this to be owned by all the seniors and not just dependent on Lisa.

3. We wanted to engage staff more at night, and make sure this was a 24-hour approach and not just something that happened during the day.

4. We wanted intentionally to work much closer with faith communities, and with two churches in particular, to expand the opportunities for people to go out and to stay connected with their faith communities. We wanted to use this as a way to extend individual time beyond two hours for some people.

5. We wanted to make sure we had a stronger focus on communication charts and decision-making agreements, and to start doing more of those.

6. We wanted to look at group activities based on one-page profiles.

7. We wanted to look at how we could support people to be greater members of their community, and to start by mapping out where they were going at the moment.

8. We wanted to explore other ways of getting people out and about more, and to see how we could involve volunteers.

9. We wanted to introduce Working Together for Change when we'd done the person-centred reviews, as a way of everybody contributing to what happened next.

As we had six months to work together on these, we thought about where we wanted to be with each one of them in six months' time and developed a project plan based on this. This gave us new success indicators, so we also updated our dashboard to reflect them.

Chapter summary: Asking where we are so we can move on

We'd put our project into effect, and seen some dramatic changes both in the lives of the people living at Bruce Lodge, and in the working practices and principles of the staff. But we knew that we needed to make sure these changes would last, and that we could do more and better.

So we asked ourselves four questions: What have we tried? What have we learnt? What were we pleased about? And what were we concerned about? We found out that the changes we'd observed were real, and that individuals and their families really appreciated the work we'd done. The staff did too. We also found out about some glitches that we needed to sort out, and some bigger concerns about making the project sustainable and wider ranging in the future.

This led us to our final question: What were we going to do next? We took ideas from the staff and the leadership team, and set ourselves ten goals for the final six months of the project.

In the next chapter we look at what we did to meet these goals.

7

Night Staff, Volunteers and Faith Communities

HELEN

Helen (see Figure 7.1) is wonderful company because she has so many stories to tell. She loves deep conversation and will debate anything, particularly current affairs. She loves to get out and about, and says it means the world to her. Anything and anywhere, she's interested in everything, and she must be busy.

Helen was born in 1929. Her late dad, Charles, is incredibly important to her – she doesn't speak about her late husband. Her dad was a vet in the Army and he treated injured horses: the book *War Horse* is important to Helen as it is the story of a wounded horse, which obviously reminds her of her father's work. Animals, and particularly horses, are a great love of Helen's: they always have been and still are to this day.

When we met with Helen and her family, one of the things she wanted to try during her individual time each month was going out to the local café in the park to see the animals. Helen loves dogs, and the thought of having a dog to look after would be wonderful. Helen spends lots of time in her room as, although she's a very outgoing woman, she chooses to stay there.

Lynn, her daughter, and her son-in-law Matthew are very important to Helen. They live in Dubai. Lynn visits approximately every six weeks and spends lots of time with her mum. She tells her mum how the four grandchildren – Josh, Tim, Lucy and Emily, who mean so much to Helen – are doing.

One of the things we learned was that Helen doesn't choose to be in large groups for too long as she finds it quite overwhelming. We wanted to help her make her room as homely as possible, so that her bedroom door is like her front door. In this way, if she chooses to leave her room, it's to go to the communal parts of the building for a particular purpose or to join something, in the same way as if we were going out of our front door, it would be to go out somewhere.

We wanted to build with Helen on this idea of her bedroom being her room where she spends her time and to encourage her to join in communal activity so that she doesn't become isolated, with not many people around her. This is something the staff are working hard on.

This is how Helen's daughter Lynn describes what has changed for her mum:

My name is Lynn Perkin. My mum has been a resident here in Bruce Lodge since October 2012. But because I live abroad in Dubai, it's critical for me to feel she's in a safe and nurturing environment.

A very nice woman called Gill came in and interviewed both myself and my mum (my husband happened to be there at the same time). We talked about what had made Mum's life happy before she came into the residential care, and what things were important to her and to us as a family.

Mum is not a very gregarious person and not terribly good in big group events. But she's responded well to this one-to-one set-up that's going on here at Bruce Lodge. That's very valuable to me – again, who's so far away – to know somebody is taking a special interest in her, because I hate to think of her as being left out or alone a lot of the time. So it's great and it's working very well.

Clearly one of the major things for us, with me living so far away, is that contact is important – not just phone calls, but perhaps visual contact. And we were able to achieve that by setting up a Skype scenario via the computer. This was very alien to Mum, but the staff helped her sit at the computer, so that's a great step forward for us.

During this visit we had a Skype conversation with my husband. He walked the computer around our house in Dubai and showed Mum a little of the environment we live in, and that was really valuable to see. It feels so much closer than a telephone call, and works very well.

Hopefully it will also enable our four children, who are dotted all over the place, to make occasional Skype calls to their granny. I feel it's important to keep that visual stimulus up, so that hopefully she can retain her memories of us for even longer.

We talked about her love of animals. As I said, Mum's not a terribly gregarious person, but she does enjoy one-to-one contact. She's still quite physically fit and loves to get out. Mum is matched to someone who loves dogs and who takes Mum dog-walking.

Also to my amazement, the staff have managed to get Mum out swimming. She's 83 and to my knowledge has never been to a swimming pool before, so that's an amazing achievement.

> *I was phoned by a member of staff asking if I could provide some monies for Mum to have a swimming costume. I was a little amazed at this and said 'Well, I don't think my mum swims. She doesn't swim.' They said, 'Oh, we asked her and she was very keen to go.'*
>
> *I naturally encouraged that, and we discussed it before she went. I said 'It may well be that she declines to go in the water when she gets there.' But we all felt it was good for her to get out and about, even if she just sat on the side at the end of the pool.*
>
> *I believe she had a rubber ring and floated around quite happily, and thoroughly enjoyed the experience. And she has said she's looking forward to going again.*

Moving into the second phase

From the four plus one questions we described in Chapter 6, we had a fresh focus. We wanted to communicate what we were doing through photos on a community map and in people's rooms; to extend people's hours through links with faith communities and volunteers; to extend what we were doing to night time and to do everything we could to embed and make the process we had begun into a habit.

Sharing photos

We wanted a way for everyone who lives, works or visits Bruce Lodge to see what people were doing and where they were going during their individual time. We created a large map of the area around Bruce Lodge, printed out photos of people using their individual time and linked them to the map with wool. The first version looked a bit rough and ready, but it was a start!

What is important to Helen

- Lynn her daughter and son in law Matthew, Josh, Tim, Lucy and Emily her grandchildren.
- Speaking with Lynn and Matthew on Skype each week as they are based in Dubai.
- Seeing Lynn six times weekly when she comes to the UK to see mum.
- Matthew's mum, Jean, visiting.
- Doing her daily exercises, being independent – "if I can do it myself I will do".
- Doing her hair – putting her rollers in and going to the hairdresser each week.
- Helen loves reading – history or stories about animals are her favourite. Helen will tell you she has never been a lover of thrillers or romances.
- Her late dad Charles, talking about him – dad was a vet in the army.
- Animals, horses especially have always been a great love of Helen's and still are.
- Deep conversation – "about anything" current affairs are a topic Helen loves a good debate about!
- Poetry has always meant a lot to Helen.
- "Getting out and about means the world to me – anything and anywhere, I am interested in everything!"
- "I must be busy".
- TV isn't of great interest though Helen enjoys 'Strictly' and 'Songs of praise'.
- Having a Sunday newspaper delivered for a good read.
- Her Roman Catholic faith.

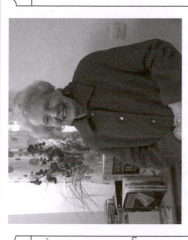

Helen

What those who know Helen best say they like and admire about her

Very interesting conversationalist.

Kind and generous lady.

Wonderful company.

Sense of humour.

A tireless worker/endlessly active.

Devotion to those she loves whether human or animal.

How we can best support Helen

- Know that Helen does not choose to be in large groups for too long, she finds it overwhelming.
- Helen will clean her own room and do her own hand washing – check in with her if she needs anything.
- Helen is fiercely independent, be mindful that she will be reluctant to ask for help - so offer it.
- Support Helen to wash her hair once a week as well as ensuring she goes to the hairdresser every week.
- Be aware Helen has asked for support to have a bath each week – ensure this happens.
- Know that Helen will need support to speak with Lynn and Matthew at least weekly on Skype in terms of it being set up – see one of the senior staff team for detail around what needs to happen and when.
- One to one conversation is crucial to Helen's well being – chat with her often.

Figure 7.1 Helen's one-page profile

We asked each of the seniors to look at different ways that people could share their photos in their rooms

- Some people are making a journal together. This is what Ken does with Sarah.

- Winifred has a digital frame in her room that includes photos of her and Beryl having coffee breaks and working together.

- Helen has a collage of photos in her room, which is a great talking point, for staff and family.

Seniors taking the lead

This felt like the make-or-break action for us. Could we support the seniors, some of whom were new in post, to feel the same commitment and show the same leadership as Lisa?

The first step was to help the seniors really understand what was expected, what their core responsibilities were, and where they could use their own judgement and experiment. Gill suggested using the person-centred thinking tool called 'the doughnut' for this. Working with Lisa and Kerri they identified core responsibilities for all of the seniors, and ones that were specific to their roles.

These are the roles they identified:

Joy: group activities and working with faith communities

Maz: different ways of sharing photos in people's rooms

Karen and Kerri: community mapping and keeping the map up to date with how people were using their time

Val: staff one-page profiles – keeping these updated and adding new ones when staff joined

Sue: night-time one-page profiles.

All seniors were responsible for making sure that the learning logs were reviewed and that the one-page profiles were updated from the learning logs.

Gill and Lisa thought about how Lisa could use her supervision time with each senior to look at what was working and not working in their roles, and to support them to celebrate success and solve problems. One of the responsibilities that they had was to build up the number of communication charts and decision-making agreements so that eventually everyone would have them. Gill provided initial coaching and support around this.

A 24-hour approach: Night staff

This goal was seen as one of the most ambitious ones by the leadership team, who spent a whole meeting thinking about the role of night staff in relation to personalisation. Gill and Lisa had checked that all of the night staff had a one-page profile.

First, we thought about night staff and what their role was and could be. What if night staff saw their role as being sleep experts, and were skilled at helping people to get the best night's sleep possible?

If we wanted to do this, then we would need to learn how to support each person to have the best night's sleep. So we developed night-time one-page profiles.

These were the headings that we used:

- what support the person needs to get to sleep

- if the person wakes up during the night, how to help him/ her get back to sleep

- if the person wakes up early, what you need to know or do.

We asked two of the enthusiastic night staff, Lewis and Janet, to try these out for us, to see if the headings worked.

We were considering how Marie was feeling about the life she was living and the support she was receiving. Something else she was really struggling with was finding the bathroom, particularly at night time, when staff noticed that she became disorientated on getting out of bed.

It was clear that particular things needed to be in place for Marie at night. If Marie wants to use the bathroom during the night she must put her slippers on. If she can't find them she'll get more and more upset as she searches, and that makes it more unlikely she'll be able to settle back to sleep. Marie will find the toilet much more easily if the bathroom light is on, and seeing the toilet is a clue that helps her locate it.

Marie must have plenty of tissues in her bathroom, because she must always blow her nose after using the toilet and she won't go back to bed until she's done this. So there was some very crucial information that staff, particularly at night, needed to know.

Something else we learned was that although Marie generally sleeps well (usually only waking to go to the toilet), if she does wake early it's probably because she's cold. So she'll really appreciate us leaving her jumper at the bottom of the bed, so that if she wakes she can put it on. Otherwise, she'll get up and search for her jumper, and again that makes it less likely that she'll be able to get back to sleep.

Lewis captured this information into a night-time one-page profile for Marie, with the important information about what support she needs to get to sleep.

Night staff now know how important it is that she has her slippers, and to make sure that she has a jumper at the end of her bed. Marie's sleep has really improved. At night they now know her en-suite toilet light must be left on, that her slippers are always right beside her bed, and a walking frame is always very close by.

Activities programme

We spent time in a leadership team meeting developing ideas for a new activities programme based on everyone's one-page profile.

We looked at everyone's one-page profile, and at what was important to each person. We listed all the things from the one-page profiles that could be done in a group, and where an activity was important to more than one person. This gave a list of potential activities that were important to people who live at Bruce Lodge, and ones that other people may be interested in trying too. There was no bingo, or arts and crafts at all.

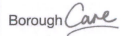 **Support at Night for … Marie**

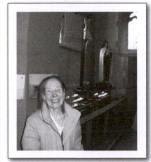

What support Marie needs to get to sleep

- Ensure Marie's en-suite light is left on.
- Her slippers must be by her bed and her walking frame within easy reach, so Marie feels secure when in bed knowing they are there.

If Marie wakes up during the night, how to help her get back to sleep

- Marie wakes to use the bathroom during the night but must first put her slippers on. If she cannot find them she will become more and more upset as she searches, making it unlikely that she will be able to settle back to sleep.
- Marie will find the toilet easily if the bathroom light is on and seeing the toilet is a cue that helps her locate it. Ensure Marie has plenty of tissues in her bathroom as she must blow her nose after using the toilet and will not return to bed until she has done this.
- Noise will upset Marie and stop her sleeping; always speak very gently with her.

If Marie wakes early, what you need to know or do

- Marie generally sleeps well, waking only to go to the bathroom. If she does wake early it is usually because she is cold. Marie really feels the cold – even during warm spells; she will get up and search for a jumper to put on. Always leave a jumper at the bottom of her bed, she will find it and put it on if she is cold.

Figure 7.2 Marie's one-page profile for night-time support

One of the seniors, Joy, developed our list into a weekly activity programme. Using this approach, people living with dementia at Bruce Lodge had an opportunity to do more of what was important to them, or try new activities that other people already enjoyed.

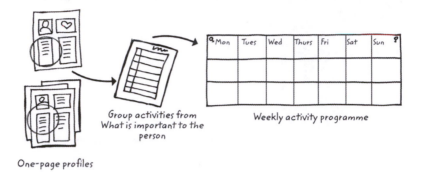

One-page profiles

Group activities from What is important to the person

Weekly activity programme

Figure 7.3 Developing the activities programme from one-page profiles

Working with volunteers

When we started working together at Bruce Lodge, Lisa was used to having students on placement, but there were no volunteers. We wanted to think differently about how we could work with 'dementia friends',[1] and specifically how volunteers could help us to extend the number of hours of individual time available to people living at Bruce Lodge. We spent time at the leadership team meeting thinking about how we could do this. This is what we came up with:

- We would need a lead person responsible for volunteers and agreed that this would be the deputy manager Kerri.

- Potential volunteers would be introduced to Bruce Lodge and have the usual information that volunteers get (Borough Care had a volunteers' policy and information).

- If, after this, they confirmed that they wanted to be a volunteer, we would support them to do their one-page profile first (whilst they were waiting for their Disclosure

---

1   Dementia Friends are volunteers who support people with dementia in the UK, www.dementiafriends.org.uk.

and Barring Service (DBS) checks (previously CRB checks) to be completed).

- The purpose of doing their one-page profile was twofold. The first was to be able to match them with someone who shared their interests who lived at Bruce Lodge. The second was to learn how to support them well as a volunteer.

In essence we were doing the matching process of volunteer and individual the other way round. This time it was based on the one-page profile of the volunteer, to find their interests and passions, and to see who in Bruce Lodge shared these. Ideally we wanted to find two or three potential matches for the volunteer, so that the person themselves and the volunteer could meet each other and find the best match that way. This would be a slightly different process each time, depending on the potential matches.

The first volunteer was Andy. Andy is matched with Helen. Andy brought his daughter Laura to the Bruce Lodge family day in the summer, and now Laura volunteers as well.

Every six months, the deputy, Kerri, is planning to have coffee and cake with all the volunteers, as a thank you and to see what is working and not working from their perspective.

Working with faith communities

Our approach to volunteering was designed directly to increase the amount of individual time that people had, through matching them to a volunteer as well as having their dedicated two hours with a member of staff a month.

The idea behind our working with faith communities was to see if we could find a way for people to feel connected and get more involved in their church or place of worship. We wanted to see if we could get to a point where people from the same church or place of worship could eventually feel confident enough to support the person to attend without staff. This would mean that they could have two hours of staff time in addition to being part of their faith community, as people from the church would take them instead of staff doing this. It would, therefore, increase the amount of individual time people had each month.

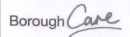

Laura's one-page profile to be a dementia friend

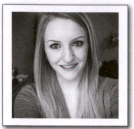

What people appreciate about me

Smart, determined, loyal, ambitious, kind, organised

What's important to me...

- My cat Sunny
- Spending time with my 'Big' family (Grand-parents, Aunties, Uncles and Cousins)
- Eating chocolate everyday
- Tea – my favourite is Builder's Brew. I like my tea strong, with milk, about 4 cups a day
- Watching TV most days, especially Desperate Housewives, The Big Bang Theory, How I Met your Mother, Pretty Little Liars
- Having time to myself, every day, especially when I come home from school
- Working hard at school at subjects I like (not homework – work hard enough at school)
- Thinking and planning my future (my career, living in Australia)
- Reading (favourites at the moment – Harry Potter series, Twilight Saga, The Book theif)
- My iPhone – particularly for the music, having it with me all the time
- Shopping and buying new clothes, to the Trafford Centre when I can afford it
- Going on holiday abroad to hot places

If I could I would...

- Travel with my friends
- Go to Glastonbury or another music festival every year
- Be a dentist or entrepreneur
- Live in Australia when I grow up
- Go to university

How best to support me as a volunteer

- Have all the information I need
- To match me with an individual or with tasks I feel I can do confidently
- Contact me by text
- Know who to speak to if I have any problems
- To be able to come twice a month at weekends or after school

Figure 7.4 Laura's volunteer one-page profile

Marie is a great example of why this is both important and possible. How could we support Marie to become a valued and contributing member of her faith community without relying solely on paid support? As Marie is very quiet, and can easily become invisible, we began to think about how we could support her to build friendships with other people at church, with a view to those people, we hoped, becoming friends and picking her up and going to church together without paid support. We wanted Marie to be able to join in more of the social events at church as well as Mass. We knew that there were other people at Bruce Lodge whose faith was important to them, so we hoped that our experience with Marie would help them too.

We spent time over two leadership team meetings thinking about this. First of all we mapped out the local churches and places of worship in the area. We thought about who we knew who was already connected – did we know families or staff who attended? What did we know about the leadership at that faith community? It was very helpful to have Chris as part of our leadership team: as a lay minister himself, he provided good insights and suggestions about people he was connected to and good ways to approach church communities.

We looked at the one-page profiles of the people who lived at Bruce Lodge to find out how many people had faith as something that was important to them. There were seven people and among them were Roman Catholics, members of the Church of England and a Jehovah's Witness. We had a big discussion about car insurance if a volunteer from the church were happy to take or collect someone, and when and if someone would need a CRB (now DBS) check.

We identified the local Kingdom Hall, a local Roman Catholic church and a local Church of England church as places to start. We thought that these would have the most potential as through the mapping process that we did they were the most local and had the greatest number of existing connections. Tim is a Eucharistic minister who visits Bruce Lodge on a weekly basis, and we asked him for his advice as well

We decided to start by talking to ministers of the churches individually and asking them to think about how to involve people in their churches. Rather than suggesting answers, we wanted to work together to see what was possible. One of the ministers suggested that we put something in the church newsletter. He did this two weeks later. Nothing has come of it so far.

We know that this is a long journey. How can we help faith communities to become dementia-friendly places that truly welcome people with dementia? How can we connect with faith communities and make the investment that this needs without more time to make this happen?

At the moment we are supporting people like Marie, who chose to spend their individual hours to go to Mass, and looking out for potential connections whilst there. We are also looking at whether a Community Circle is an approach that could help to get people from faith communities directly involved in people's lives.

Community Circles

Community Circles started in Stockport to find ways for circles of support to be available to many people, including people with dementia. A circle is a group of friends and family who meet every month to six weeks with the person. Each circle has a specific focus and purpose, chosen by the person, and is supported by a facilitator.

We wanted to see if this approach would work for Marie, to help her to become a greater part of her church community. Gill volunteered to be the facilitator for Marie's community circle, and she is being supported by Michelle from Community Circles.

The first step was to do a detailed relationship map with Marie, to look at who she knows at church already, to see where there are potential connections, and who could be invited to join her circle.

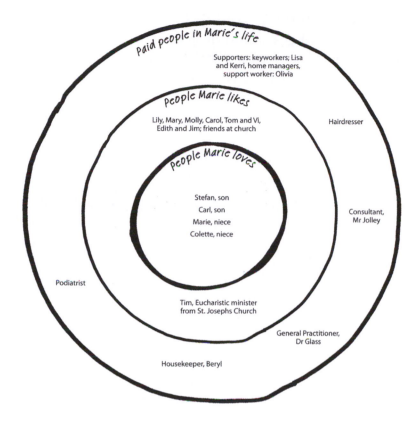

Figure 7.5 Marie's relationship circle

From this relationship map, Gill and Marie thought about who would be the best people to approach to see if they would join Marie's circle. This is where we are up to at the time of going to press.

We are hoping that specifically inviting one or two individuals who already know Marie to spend time with us working out what we can do together will enable us to make some progress. If we do establish a circle for Marie, this could then give us a way to have further conversations about the other people from Bruce Lodge who would like to be better connected to the church, and to go from there.

Chapter summary: Taking the next steps

We'd asked ourselves some searching questions as we reached the end of the first phase of our project. We found out that we were doing well: our work was giving the people at Bruce Lodge time and choices that simply weren't there before.

We also found some things we needed to do better, so Phase 2 of the project focused on these:

- We used photos to tell everyone at Bruce Lodge about the activities people had been pursuing in their individual time.

- We made the responsibilities of senior staff clearer so that key tasks were completed.

- We extended our work to the night staff and looked at how we could improve people's sleep.

- We remembered the importance of group activities and developed new ones based on the interests people had shared in the one-page profiles.

- We found ways that volunteers could extend people's individual time, and began to make links with churches in the hope that they too would voluntarily help people to take part in the life of their faith. We began to explore whether a community circle could help someone to take part in their church's life, or other activities that were important to them.

The success of a project like this lies in getting the detail right – but also in being able to see the bigger picture. In the next chapter we look at how we went on to use the lessons from person-centred reviews to inform strategic planning for the future of personalisation at Bruce Lodge and beyond.

8

Person-Centred Reviews and Working Together for Change

MARIE

Marie's initial meeting to gather the information for her one-page profile happened in February 2013. In July 2013, we again met with Marie and her family to have a person-centred review meeting. We looked at some of the things that were working and not working for Marie, and developed ways of addressing any problems. We've described below the things that weren't working, and what we did to address them.

Going to church

One of the outcomes from the meeting we had in January was the way Marie was going to spend her time. What was really important to her was her Roman Catholic faith, so she was going to be supported to go to Mass once a month. This began quite soon after that first meeting, and Marie began going to St Joseph's Church with Olivia, with whom she had been matched.

What we wanted to do next was to really build on supporting Marie to become a valued and contributing member of a faith community, and to develop friendships there so she wasn't relying solely on paid support.

We learned at Marie's review meeting that she wasn't going to Mass and church events every week. She had always belonged to St Vincent de Paul, so we decided that Olivia would speak with the chair of the St Vincent de Paul Society at St Joseph's to explore the possibility of one of the members of the Society getting to know Marie really well. We hoped that the Society member would support Marie to go to meetings with a view to making more friends who would be able to call for her each Sunday morning so she could go to Mass.

So after the review we were looking to extend the number of people who weren't paid in Marie's life so that she could go to Mass more regularly, and be much more a part of the church community in terms of all the social events that were happening. And this was a really big thing for Marie.

Poetry

Marie loves poetry (Patience Strong's poetry books are very special to her) and we learned at the review that she wasn't having the opportunity to listen to her poetry, and staff weren't able to find the time to sit and read poetry to her.

The team thought about this and decided that Sue and Marie would go to the local library and bookstores to try and find some audiobooks by Marie's favourite poets that she could listen to.

Moving around

We also learnt, because Marie's niece told us, that Marie was struggling more and more to open the doors and get around the building with a walking frame that seemed to be very cumbersome.

We had some discussion around this and decided that Kerri, the deputy manager, would make a referral for an occupational therapy assessment to consider other walking aids that may be less cumbersome than Marie's walking frame so she can get about more freely.

Marie's circle

Another action that came from the review meeting was a response to Marie clearly saying that she missed getting out and about and watching what was going on in the world. She'd already said that she wanted to be much more involved in church. So Gill would explore how to develop a circle with Marie to bring more people into her life who are not paid and who can support her to get out and about.

After the review

Lisa updated Marie's one-page profile from the new learning we'd gained during the person-centred review meeting, and made sure that it was shared with all staff.

The person-centred review meeting was a more formal way for us all to sit back down together and think with Marie about how things were going, and to identify anything we needed to add to what's important to Marie on her one-page profile. Are there new things we've learned around how best to support Marie from her perspective? How can we enhance or build on the things that are working well for Marie? And what actions do we need to take to change the things that are not working for Marie?

Person-centred reviews

Everyone has a person-centred review every six months. The review echoes a lot of the initial meeting, when we started the person's one-page profile and how they wanted to use their individual time.

The person-centred review meeting includes the individual themselves, their family, the manager, and the person who has been supporting the individual with their individual time.

It takes about an hour and a half. At the meeting we reflect together on what is working and not working from different perspectives. We look at what we can do to build on what's working and make sure it continues, and how to change what's not working and stop it from happening.

At this meeting we also review the individual time that the person chose six months ago, and any actions that came from what is working and not working.

From the person-centred review we:

- update the one-page profile with information and other changes that the person wants

- have a new understanding about what's working and not working from different perspectives

- have actions to change what's not working and to build on what is working

- have a new or updated outcome for the person's individual time.

Finally, at the end of the meeting, if the person can tell us directly themselves – and if not, we ask their family, the staff and manager – we ask them to identify the top two things that are working for them, the top two things that are not working and the top two things the person would like to do in the future. This information directly informs how Bruce Lodge continues to develop its whole approach to working with people with dementia, by using a process called Working Together for Change.

Working Together for Change

Working Together for Change (WTFC) is an eight-stage process designed to take information from person-centred reviews and use it to inform strategic planning. At Bruce Lodge we took the first 12 person-centred reviews that we did and held a day to use the WTFC process to see what those reviews were telling us about what was working and not working for people overall, and what people wanted to do in the future.

From now on, every year WTFC will take place at Bruce Lodge to look at the information from everybody who has had a person-centred review. WTFC will use that information to inform the future planning for implementing personalisation and other ongoing development.

There's also an opportunity to carry out this process not just for a single care home (in this case Bruce Lodge) but also to aggregate the information from all of the care homes across Borough Care, and use it to inform strategic business planning on an annual basis.

We think this is the clearest and the best way that individuals who are living with dementia and using the services at Bruce Lodge can directly inform how their service develops, and can contribute to the business planning for the whole of Borough Care. WTFC means that strategic plans can be created without using focus groups, and without using questionnaires, but rather by taking the information directly from what people supported by Borough Care are saying about their lives in their person-centred reviews.

Our WTFC day was the final day that the leadership team met. We invited a guest as well – the person at Stockport Council who was taking a lead on the implementation of direct payments in residential care – so that she could see how the process was working and consider how it could be used more widely across the Council.

What our Working Together for Change day revealed

Lisa brought the anonymised information from the 12 person-centred reviews, and this was written on coloured cards.

WHAT IS WORKING FOR PEOPLE

We started by looking at what people had said in their review was working for them. We clustered all of the cards onto one of the pinboards. The process for doing this simply involved the facilitator (in this case) reading out from each card one statement about what's working from the perspective of somebody who uses the services. The whole group decided where that statement goes, and whether it's clustered with other ones that have a similar theme, or whether it's a separate issue.

Once we'd done a cluster analysis on the board, we named each of the clusters and gave them headings that reflected the content of what people had said, phrased as an 'I' statement.

We established eight themes from what people told us was working in their lives:

1. I am having more conversations and being listened to.

2. I am choosing what I do.

3. I am supported by staff who know me well.

4. I am doing something that feels useful.

5. I am reconnecting with people in my community.

6. I am doing more things that I enjoy.

7. I choose who to support and who supports me.

8. I am going out and doing things I want to do.

It was brilliant to see all those statements in front of us, and everyone shared their reflections. There aren't many formal opportunities to celebrate the changes that we're making in people's lives and the difference they're telling us the changes are achieving, so it was a really good thing to do this. We then took a deep breath…and went on to do the same with the 'not working' cards.

WHAT IS NOT WORKING FOR PEOPLE

We used the same process with people's statements about what was not working. Here are the nine clusters of what people said weren't working in their lives:

1. I am less able to do things.

2. I am in poor physical health and cannot get out.

3. I don't get out as often as I want.

4. I don't always have enough money to do what I want.

5. I have important things that get lost.

6. I feel isolated when I'm having bed rest.

7. Sometimes I don't know what's happening.

8. I have no friends outside the home.

9. I miss being part of church life.

We then gave everybody an opportunity to reflect on what this told us. There are some statements that we can't change directly as they are part of people's experience of living with dementia. But there are some things that we *can* do more about. In particular, where people are less able to do things, are in poor physical health and can't get out, and sometimes don't know what's happening, there are things we can do to support them and make sure they are in the best physical health possible.

We asked everyone to vote on the clusters where we could make a difference, and to vote on their priorities for changing. Here are the ones that got the top votes:

• I have no friends outside the home.

• I miss being part of church life.

• Sometimes I don't know what's happening.

• I don't get out as often as I want.

WHAT PEOPLE WANT IN THE FUTURE

Before we started to look at action planning, we clustered the things that would be important to people in the future. This gave us eight different themes, and here is what people said they wanted:

1. I want to have a dog.

2. I want to get outside as much as possible.

3. I want to know what's happening next.

4. I want to have more company.

5. I want to stay active and busy.

6. I want to stay well and on my feet.

7. I want to be involved in the church community more regularly.

8. I want Bruce Lodge to be my home until I die.

These are very powerful and in many ways sobering statements. You can see what's important in the future also reflects both what's working and what's not working for people.

We saw strong themes resulting from several people wanting to be part of their church community; not wanting to be lonely and wanting to have more company; wanting to get out and about as much as possible; and wanting to maintain their health, stay well, and be on their feet.

In the same way as we did with the 'not working' board, we gave everybody sticky dots to vote with and told them to vote on these themes so that we could make sure we prioritised them as we went forward with the action planning.

The top themes the group voted on were:

- I want to have more company.

- I want to be involved in the church community more regularly.

- I want to get outside as much as possible.

We had a big conversation about the individual who wanted to have a dog and we'll talk more about that later on in this chapter.

By now we had clustered all the information from what was working, not working and important in the future. We'd identified the themes people were telling us about based on the information from their person-centred reviews. We prioritised the themes to take forward into actions, and these were the 'not working' ones we decided to work on:

- I feel isolated when I'm having bed rest.

- I have no friends outside the home.

- I don't get out as often as I want.

- I miss being part of church life.

- I want to have a dog.

From clusters to root causes and success

For each of these 'not working' themes we then used a process called 'five whys' to identify the possible reasons for something not to be working. This was very important so that we didn't make a knee-jerk reaction by going straight to action planning without first taking time to really understand why something was not working for people.

We got our heads together and did some mind-mapping of possible reasons. Then we went from potential reasons to what success looked like. We looked at success from different perspectives. Here is an example around one of the priorities – people feeling isolated when they are on bed rest.

'I FEEL ISOLATED WHEN I'M HAVING BED REST.'
Possible root causes

- Staff are confusing bed rest with people wanting to be alone, so they're automatically leaving people alone when they're bed resting.

- Visitors might be doing the same as well (leaving people alone, and not booking visiting time when people are on bed rest).

- The door might be closed, so people don't naturally pop in when people are on bed rest.

- Bed rest always happens in the bedroom.

- Staff don't explore other places where it might be possible for people to be physically resting and horizontal, but also engaged with other people.

Success from different perspectives

People: 'I have company when I'm on bed rest.'

Staff: 'We know people are happy, well and safe, and have company when they're on bed rest.'

Stockport Council: 'We know that people on bed rest have company, and their needs are being met.'

From our understanding about why this might be happening (possible root causes) and what we wanted to achieve (success from different perspectives) we could identify potential actions.

Action planning

Here are some of the actions that we wanted to explore:

- Talk to family members about visiting specifically when people are on bed rest.

- When we get volunteers or students, focus them on people who are on bed rest and make sure that they have company if they want it.

- Look at digital photos and audio books and other ways that people could perhaps be more engaged when they're on bed rest.

- Have conversations with district nurses about whether there are different ways that we can make sure people are getting bed rest, but can also be in places where they can have company with others.

We turned these into specific and measurable actions with someone responsible, and used the same process for each of the prioritised five actions we wanted to work on.

A dog?
Looking at both root causes and success from different perspectives led to very interesting discussions and debates, like the ones we had around someone having a dog.

We explored whether it was possible for one individual to own a dog and be responsible for looking after it, and what that would look like in terms of other people getting involved in looking after the dog. It was good to explore this from what the Local Authority would see as acceptable, what the staff would worry about and the potential implications for other people who lived in the home.

If we had not used Working Together for Change, these conversations would be unlikely to have taken place. There is now an action plan to explore what could be possible around having a dog, reflecting different concerns, but wanting to explore all options as well.

Phase 3
The Working Together for Change process gave us the actions for Phase 3 of our project. The first phase of work we did together was determined by the leadership team, and was to establish one-page profiles and individual time, and get them implemented within the home.

Staff were directly involved in informing Phase 2. We worked directly with staff to get their feedback about what was working and not working, and what they wanted to see covered in Phase 2, as well as continuing to pay attention to the comments cards from families and professionals. The leadership team fed this information into an analysis of what we had tried, what we had learned, what we were pleased about, what we were concerned about and what we wanted to do next in Phase 2.

Phase 3 – the new phase we were going into – was entirely directed by people who lived at Bruce Lodge and were using the service. We took the information from person-centred reviews and used the WTFC process to identify people's priorities, to keep what was working and change what was not working, and to move closer to what they wanted to see in the future. We decided we should stop talking about phases now! This was going to become the way that Bruce Lodge developed and changed – by learning from what is working and not working for people through their person-centred reviews, and using this Working Together for Change process to determine priorities for change.

Can you go further than that? We think so.

A further step would be to ask staff at their annual appraisal what is working and not working from their perspective, and to use the Working Together for Change process with this information. This has to be so much better than a staff satisfaction survey. One care home for older people in the South West has already successfully used this approach.

You could go further still, and at the person-centred review ask people for the top two things that are working and not working from the families' perspective as well, and the two things that they would like to see in the future.

Working Together for Change would then be about looking at these three perspectives – from people who live at Bruce Lodge, staff and families – and setting priorities for change that reflect what matters to people who live there and take into account what matters to staff and families too.

9

Overall Impact and Lessons Learned

What difference has personalisation made?

Lisa, the manager at Bruce Lodge, will tell you that the benefits of the approaches we have used during this personalisation project have been:

> *Just incredible: matching individuals and staff around shared interests has been a real win-win: for the person, doing something that matters to them with someone who is enthusiastic about it, and for the staff, having an opportunity to share a hobby or interest at work.*

The benefits have been huge for individuals and their families too. Lisa shares a comment from Maureen, the daughter of Winifred who lives in the home:

> *Mum can be heard singing aloud as she carries out the chores she did so routinely in her own home before she moved here. She is happier, chatting more, using fuller sentences, is sleeping better and generally more alive.*

Winifred's story is just one example of the difference made in the lives of people you have learned about in this book. Sometimes it's about living in the moment, or having a purpose to get out of bed in the morning, or being active members of the community. This is a long way from the stereotypical idea of people living with dementia – and this is part of the change we are seeing at Bruce Lodge.

Our quality of life is determined by the presence or the absence of those things that are important to us and so we have clearly taken this into account at Bruce Lodge.

Working and living together

Team members say they feel they know each other much better as a result of developing the one-page profiles. They have different conversations based on what they have learned about each other and therefore have become a closer team, and they are much clearer about what good support looks like to each other. Lisa, the manager, also said she is much clearer about what good support looks like to individual staff members and she has improved supervision sessions, team meetings, and the way the team work together and with individuals as a result.

Choosing the right person to provide support during individual time was arguably one of the most important decisions that made a difference to people living at Bruce Lodge – doing something we want to do can still be a miserable experience if we are not with someone we like. Using the one-page profiles of staff or volunteers and people living at Bruce Lodge was key to ensuring people had the best possible experience during their individual time because it meant they had a say in who they spent time with and were supported by.

Real personalisation requires a cultural change from a task-focused ethos to one that values what matters most to the people being supported. Being able to deliver this support in the way that individuals want it, according to their one-page profiles, means this cultural change has clearly been embraced by all at Bruce Lodge. Staff do not simply use the vocabulary but naturally involve people in tasks, and so living and working at Bruce Lodge has become a shared experience. Staff no longer wear uniforms and there is little sense of a 'them and us' culture: people living at Bruce Lodge are respectfully perceived as being the experts in their own lives.

Staff are going the extra mile in demonstrable ways, thinking about the people living at Bruce Lodge even when not at work. For example, the housekeeper Roy looked for some of his old classical CDs as he knew John who lived at Bruce Lodge also enjoyed that genre of music. Roy set John up with the CDs playing in a small lounge where he wouldn't be disturbed and then went about his work, popping back in to see how John was enjoying the music now and again.

A deeper understanding

The staff team are reporting really positive results, with a decrease in perceived challenging behaviour due to their increased recognition that they have to seek out the feeling that lies beneath the behaviour. They now try to understand what people are actually communicating to them through their behaviour and to explore how they can support people well in response.

People are seen as individuals and get individualised support. Staff morale is high as everybody at the home takes responsibility for driving up standards and putting the person at the centre of everything that happens. Staff are able to describe numerous examples of increased well-being occurring during individual time and also on a day-to-day basis: one-page profiles are used as job descriptions that ensure people get more of what is important to them, so those things that increase well-being are consistently supported regardless of the number of staff involved in providing that support.

The approach we've described in this book has affected each person at Bruce Lodge's day-to-day experience, making it more likely it is how they want it to be.

A new culture

Staff are describing their approach as 'simply the way we work'. They are thinking differently about the way they present how people are using their time. For example, Ceri has a digital photo frame, a number of people have photo albums, Molly has a collage of photos over her door, and there is a community map in the foyer area of the home where people often gather; all of these encourage conversation amongst staff, people living at Bruce Lodge, family members and visitors about the different things people are doing when they are in the community. Work continues to expand on how we capture the things people are doing and share them in ways that make sense for each person.

The activity programme also looks totally different as each group activity is designed around the individuals taking part, reflecting what is important to them and led by a staff member who also has an interest in that activity. For example, groups now take part in baking and Bible sessions.

Better night-times

Another difference is that people are much better supported during the night. For example, Joe would often get up in the night and walk along the corridor, and the night staff who knew Joe well recognised that this usually meant he needed the bathroom. This was captured on the one-page profile for night-time, and even new night staff would know that best support meant asking him to link arms with them and guiding him to his en-suite bathroom. Once he returned to bed, staff would sit and reassure him that breakfast was not ready yet and he could go back to sleep, and this would help him settle down and go back to sleep.

Really listening

People clearly felt listened to: right through implementation we took feedback from staff, families, health professionals, volunteers and social care staff through comment cards. These were reviewed at leadership meetings monthly, and feedback was given to people who had made comments.

We held meetings with staff to ask what was working and not working from their perspective and also with families and individuals together to look at what was working and not working for them. Once we'd listened, we took action that made a difference to people living at Bruce Lodge and their allies.

We worked actively with those who loved and cared most about the people living at Bruce Lodge, listening well to the rich contribution they had to make and acknowledging the value of family members' roles in their relative's life. Asking different questions led to different conversations that gave us a thorough understanding of what was going to work for each individual. In turn this made us think differently about how support was provided. This information ensured that each person's support was tailored to their needs and aspirations – and that is the very bedrock of personalisation. We listened well to May, who is living with dementia, many months ago and made a change to the way we supported her:

> If people would ask me I can still tell them what I want. I just need a bit more help getting those things these days. I can't just go and have a

coffee in my favourite café because I may not find my way back. Life isn't worth living without those small joys so what do we do?

Overall, the project has made everyone involved feel a greater sense of connection to Bruce Lodge: staff, family members and volunteers are bringing in things to support other people's individual time; there are interesting conversations going on between all parties around who is doing what and where. Gillian, whose mum lives at Bruce Lodge, described it as 'a real buzz about the place'.

The impact for Borough Care Ltd

What was the impact for Borough Care? There was more than a 100 per cent increase in enquiries to Bruce Lodge, and over 50 per cent of these specifically mentioned the 'personalised time'.

Lynn, whose mum lives at Bruce Lodge, commented, 'It was the idea that Mum would be able to continue doing some of those things that brought her such joy, such as going to a show or to see horses that made us choose Bruce Lodge.'

There was also a positive impact on Borough Care's reputation – they were finalists in The National Dementia Awards in the innovation category. Borough Care embedded this approach into their dementia care strategy and are now extending it to the other care homes.

How did we measure the difference?

When trying a new approach, it is vital to measure its effectiveness from the very beginning. We used a range of measures to ensure that we covered all angles of the work we were doing. We used:

- The Progress for Providers self-assessment tool

- The Quality of Interactions Schedule (QUIS), an observational audit tool

- Dementia Care Mapping (DCM).

So we were really clear about the areas Bruce Lodge was strong in and the areas where further work was needed. This gave us a baseline to measure the changes that we were making. When we used each of these tools again at least 12 months later we saw significant increases in each of the baselines. We therefore had hard evidence of the improvements we were seeing day to day.

Below is a summary of the changes we saw via each of these measures.

Progress for Providers

Progress for Providers is a nationally well-regarded self-assessment tool to enable providers to check how they are doing in delivering personalised services to people living with dementia. The Care Quality Commission (CQC) are training their staff in using it, and Alistair Burns, National Clinical Director of Dementia, has endorsed it.

Progress for Providers gave us a baseline of where we were in April 2012, and how much progress we had made when we reviewed it in August 2013.

Here are the key indicators in Progress for Providers:

SECTION 1: THE PERSON

1. We see and treat the person with dementia as an individual, with dignity and respect.

2. We understand the person's history.

3. We know and act on what matters to the person.

4. We know and act on what the person wants in the future (outcomes).

5. We know and respond to how the person communicates.

6. The person is supported to make choices and decisions every day.

7. We know exactly how the person wants to be supported and how to support them to be fully part of everyday life.

8. We know what is working and not working for the person, and we are changing what is not working.

9. We support people to initiate and maintain friendships and relationships.

10. We support the person to be part of their community and civic life.

11. The environment is pleasant, homely and busy.

12. We support individuals to be in the best possible physical health.

13. There is a person-centred culture of respect and warmth.

14. People have personal possessions.

15. Meal times are pleasurable, flexible, social occasions.

SECTION 2: THE FAMILY

1. The home is a welcoming place for families.

2. Family members have good information.

3. Families contribute their knowledge and expertise.

4. We support family relationships to continue and develop.

SECTION 3: THE STAFF AND MANAGER

1. We have knowledge, skills and understanding of person-centred practices.

2. Staff are supported individually to develop their skills in using person-centred practices.

3. Our team has a clear purpose.

4. We have an agreed way of working that reflects our values.

5. Staff know what is important to each other and how to support each other.

6. Staff know what is expected of them.

7. Staff feel that their opinions matter.

8. Staff are thoughtfully matched to people and rotas are personalised to people who are supported.

9. Recruitment and selection is person centred.

10. We have a positive, enabling approach to risk.

11. Training and development is matched to staff.

12. Supervision is person centred.

13. Staff have appraisals and individual development plans.

14. Meetings are positive and productive.

The progress that a particular residential home is making towards delivering personalised support is scored against each of the above key indicators from Levels 1 to 5, reflecting the ability of organisations to offer people with dementia increased opportunity to have control of their life. Levels 1 and 2 signify that residential homes are beginning to look at and address personalisation. Levels 3 or 4 signify that residential homes are delivering person-centred care. Level 5 signifies excellence, that the home is delivering personalised support to people with dementia, including individualised funding.

Figure 9.1 demonstrates the increase in scores using Progress for Providers between initial completion in April 2012 and review in August 2013.

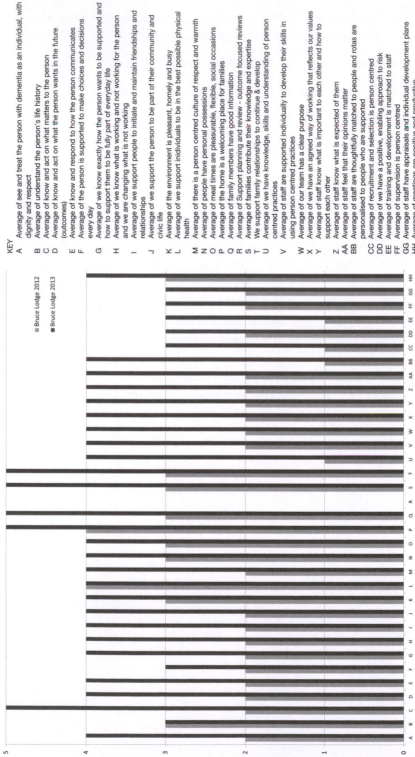

KEY

A Average of see and treat the person with dementia as an individual, with dignity and respect
B Average of understand the person's life history
C Average of know and act on what matters to the person
D Average of know and act on what the person wants in the future (outcomes)
E Average of know and respond to how the person communicates
F Average of the person is supported to make choices and decisions every day
G Average of we know exactly how the person wants to be supported and how to support them to be fully part of everyday life
H Average of we know what is working and not working for the person and we are changing what is not working
I Average of we support people to initiate and maintain friendships and relationships
J Average of we support the person to be part of their community and civic life
K Average of the environment is pleasant, homely and busy
L Average of we support inidividuals to be in the best possible physical health
M Average of there is a person centred culture of respect and warmth
N Average of people have personal possessions
O Average of meal times are pleasurable, flexible, social occasions
P Average of the home is a welcoming place for families
Q Average of family members have good information
R Average of Support planning and review - outcome focused reviews
S Average of families contribute their knowledge and expertise
T We support family relationships to continue & develop
U Average of we have knowledge, skills and understanding of person centred practices
V Average of staff are supported individually to develop their skills in using person centred practices
W Average of our team has a clear purpose
X Average of we have an agreed way of working that reflects our values
Y Average of staff know what is important to each other and how to support each other
Z Average of staff know what is expected of them
AA Average of staff feel that their opinions matter
BB Average of staff are thoughtfully matched to people and rotas are personalised to people who are supported
CC Average of recruitment and selection is person centred
DD Average of we have a positive, enabling approach to risk
EE Average of training and development is matched to staff
FF Average of supervision is person centred
GG Average of staff have appraisals and individual development plans
HH Average of meetings are positive and productive

Figure 9.1 Before and after scores for Progress for Providers

Quality of Interactions (QUIS)

QUIS aims to capture through observation the lived experience of people with dementia, living or spending time in a care setting. We carried out the QUIS observations in March 2012 and again in August 2013. QUIS captures the percentage of interactions under each of the headings in Table 9.1.

Table 9.1 QUIS observations in March 2012

Positive social	Positive care	Neutral	Negative protective	Negative restrictive
0%	17%	70%	13%	0%

Table 9.2 captures the information we gathered in August 2013. It shows marked increases in positive social and positive care interactions, and a reduction in neutral care and negative protective interactions.

Table 9.2 QUIS observations in August 2013

Positive social	Positive care	Neutral	Negative protective	Negative restrictive
17%	37%	40%	7%	0%

The increased scorings were based on observed interactions where there was a clear presence of genuine warmth being offered to individuals and lots of caring conversations were going on. Staff laughed and joked with people and there were lots of hugs between staff and people living in the home. Staff clearly felt passionate about where they worked and proud of what they provided. People were involved in activities they clearly enjoyed: two men were supported to set up a game of dominoes, a basket of freshly laundered clothes was brought to a lady who happily spent an hour folding them and another man was engaged in conversation with a volunteer about a recent outing where he had been on a boat.

Dementia Care Mapping (DCM)

DCM also aims to capture the experience of care from the standpoint of the person living with dementia. It has gained national and international recognition as a reliable evaluation tool since the late 1980s. Mapping was carried out in April 2012 and again for comparison in September 2013.

DCM captures minute by minute what the person is doing, their relative well-being, measured through their level of mood and engagement, and crucially the staff actions and inactions that may have an impact on their well-being. While we recognise that the staff actions are nearly always unintentional, they help us to understand and change the culture of care that surrounds the person.

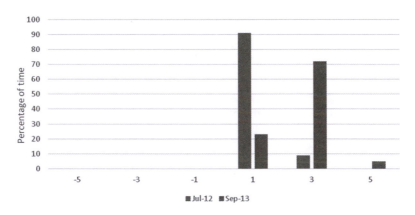

Figure 9.2 Group well-being profile

Figure 9.2 shows the difference in percentage of time that individuals spent in each of the levels of mood and engagement from the first and second observations.

This shows a significant shift away from neutral care. In July 2012 the majority of time (91%) was spent with participants showing no signs of positive or negative mood and being only briefly engaged. In September 2013, however, we see that the majority of time (72%) was spent with people showing considerable signs of either positive mood or engagement. People did still spend time in a neutral state, but the overall percentage of time spent in that state had been reduced from 91 per cent in July 2012 to just 23 per cent in September 2013.

It was great to see as well that in September 2013 people spent 4 per cent of the observed time showing very high levels of well-being.

This indicates that people are experiencing higher levels of well-being and are spending less time in a neutral or passive state.

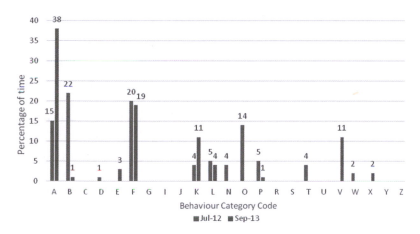

Figure 9.3 Group behaviour category grid

Figure 9.3 shows the difference in percentage of time that individuals spent engaged in different activities. In DCM we use 23 letters to indicate how a person is engaged and occupied. A full list of these can be found in the Appendix.

Some categories have a higher potential for well-being than others, as they offer a great opportunity to connect with others, or to make use of existing skills or gain new skills. The high potential categories are A, D, E, F, G, I, J, K, L, O, P, R, S, T, V, X, Y and Z.

In 2012 we saw that people spent time in 8 of the 18 high-potential categories. In 2013 we also saw them spend time in 8 of the 18 highest-potential categories, but there were significant differences. For example, in 2013 we saw considerably more independent walking (shown as K), with a rise from 4 per cent to 11 per cent of the observed time. This may indicate that people were supported more and felt more able to walk and move independently within Bruce Lodge.

The percentage of time spent in simply talking (coded as A) rose from 15 per cent in July 2012 to 38 per cent in September 2013. This indicates that, over the observed time, people were talking and connecting more with others around them.

In September 2013 people were engaged in V (work-like activity, ordinary tasks and jobs within the setting) for 11 per cent of the time. During the observations we saw people making their own sandwiches, instructing others how make a really good trifle, washing up and cleaning the tables. These are tasks and roles that might otherwise be completed by staff, rather than people living within the Home. V was not observed in July 2012.

The only medium-potential category is B, described as being in a borderline state where an individual is passively engaged in their surroundings, not taking an active part but watching others. In July 2012 we saw people in a borderline state for 22 per cent of the observed time. This dropped to just 1 per cent of the observed time in September 2013. This may indicate that staff were better skilled at drawing people into activities, and also that the activities were available was better suited to people's abilities so that they could engage more, and more often.

The lowest potential categories are those that indicate a withdrawn or distressed state. These are shown as C, U and W. It is good to see that neither C (withdrawn) nor U (unresponded to distress) were observed on either occasion. However, in July 2012, 2 per cent of the observed time was spent with individuals in W, a negative state where the person is attempting to hold themselves together and where they are seen to be engaged in repetitive, self-stimulatory actions such as rocking or wringing their hands. In September 2013, no negative states were observed.

The final set of data relates to staff interactions that either uphold a person's well-being or undermine it. These are described in DCM as 'personal enhancers' (actions that uphold well-being and personhood) or 'personal detractors' (actions that undermine a person's sense of personhood). These are grouped around the psychological needs of comfort, identity, attachment, occupation and inclusion. The tables below show the number of enhancers and detractors observed on both occasions.

Table 9.3 Personal enhancers and detractors: July 2012

Psychological need	Highly detracting	Detracting	Enhancing	Highly enhancing
Comfort		2	2	
Identity		2	2	
Attachment		0	4	
Occupation		8	5	
Inclusion		2	2	
Total	0	14	15	0

Table 9.4 Personal enhancers and detractors: September 2013

Psychological need	Highly detracting	Detracting	Enhancing	Highly enhancing
Comfort		1	2	1
Identity			1	1
Attachment			1	
Occupation			1	3
Inclusion		3	5	1
Total	0	4	10	6

The tables show that in July 2012 there were a total of 29 staff interactions that had potential for either upholding or undermining the well-being of people at Bruce Lodge. Of these, 48 per cent had the potential to undermine well-being, and 52 per cent had the potential to uphold and enhance well-being. There were no highly enhancing episodes. This is not a negative indicator, as it is not always common to see highly enhancing actions. It was good to see that there were no highly detracting episodes – those that might seriously undermine a person's well-being.

In September 2013 there were a total of 20 staff interactions that had the potential for either upholding or undermining the well-being of people at Bruce Lodge. Of these, 80 per cent had the potential to uphold and enhance well-being, and 37.5 per cent of those actions were highly enhancing to the individuals' well-being and personhood. These were wonderful snatches of time when staff were celebrating, facilitating and enabling people simply to have great fun.

Although there were still episodes where staff actions undermined well-being, at 20 per cent this is lower than the percentage observed in July 2012, when these episodes represented 48 per cent of the total. Although some old culture actions remain, such as staff talking over people, the tables indicate a significant shift towards a more inclusive, relationship-based approach where people are valued for their identity and for the gifts they bring.

But DCM is not just about numbers. It also helps us to listen in on the conversations and experiences that really make a difference to a person's day.

In one dining room, ladies – including Winnie, Jean, Doreen and May – were sitting at two tables being supported by staff to make trifles. The atmosphere was very relaxed but also very lively. Staff were sensitively supporting everyone to be involved in building their trifles. It was fantastic to see that staff were able to let go of control. As a result, we were all transported to a family kitchen with everyone gathered around the tables, gossiping, laughing, joking and teasing one another. May reached out to a member of staff as they walked past, and pulling her towards her, felt the texture of her tee-shirt before complimenting her on the colour and how much it suited her. The two then chatted briefly about preferred colours. Others at the table joined in, talking all at once about their favourite colours. As the trifles were completed Jean noticed that there was lots of whisked cream left in the bowl. She pulled it towards her and first using the spoon, and then her fingers, licked the bowl clean. A staff member standing nearby noticed what she was doing. They winked at each other and the staff member reached over to wipe her finger round the bowl to taste the cream. Both women then laughed at each other. This was evidence of genuine friendship, with both Jean and the staff member showing very great levels of well-being. This was not carer and cared for, but two friends being indulgent and colluding together against conventions.

Blanche had used her personalised time that day to visit a local garden centre, and had returned just in time for the afternoon coffee and cakes. She came into the foyer café hesitantly at first as there must have seemed to be lots of people and noise. The coffee break was well under way, music was playing, a few people were dancing arm in arm. Blanche appeared tired and uncertain. A member of staff saw her and welcomed her by calling hello and approaching with her arms spread wide. Blanche smiled and relaxed immediately. The staff member guided Blanche to a chair in the centre of the café and then sat down on the floor next to her. They held hands and chatted for a few minutes about her outing. As the staff member got up to fetch Blanche a cup of coffee, other staff waved or called over, asking about her time out and what she had had for lunch. Blanche could be seen to be in a very high state of well-being as she enjoyed being the centre of attention. After a few minutes her coffee arrived and Blanche was seen to settle down into her chair and relax, enjoying watching others in the café.

On another occasion Lily was making sandwiches in the dining room, sitting at the table with her friends. Throughout the time observed Lily called out and cajoled the staff in the room in humour. She constantly chided, laughed at comments made, and called and beckoned to them. The staff responded to every comment and both Lily and the staff shared a smile, a laugh, a kiss or a cuddle at different times. Throughout the event staff skilfully held Lily in the session by responding to her affection with genuine warmth and affirmation.

In the other dining room Doreen had tired of making the trifles and had stood to leave the table, but she hesitated as she seemed uncertain what to do next. A staff member called to her and asked if she wanted to join the others for coffee. The two joined hands, and Doreen could be seen to smile and acknowledge the staff member before they walked out into the garden towards the garden café. The walk was measured and relaxed and the two could be seen stopping very frequently as the staff member pointed to a flower or a butterfly. The two walked companionably through the garden before disappearing from view into the café. Throughout, Doreen could be seen occasionally leaning against the staff member, but always tightly holding her hand and following her gestures as she pointed out interesting things in the garden.

Conclusion

Before we started this project, we'd used Individual Service Funds with a handful of people. We'd seen the difference that this could make to people's lives, but we didn't yet know how practical it would be to apply our approach with a far larger group of people, and particularly with people who had dementia. At Bruce Lodge, we had an opportunity to find out, working with 43 people who lived there, all of whom had dementia. We had to achieve this without any additional funding, other than training and support. With only two hours a month for each person who lived at Bruce Lodge, and the dedication and commitment of the staff, and their willingness to try something completely new, we achieved some remarkable results.

In this book you may suspect we've cherry-picked the highlights – and stories like those of Winifred, whose love of life returned when she was asked to help with the housekeeping – do stand out. But there were many such stories, and over and above the individual personal stories, what we're proudest of is the cultural shift we achieved in such a short time.

Today, not only does Bruce Lodge now have ISFs well established for everyone living there, but personalisation is absolutely part of its culture. Every single person at Bruce Lodge sees themselves as part of a community, whether they live there, work there, volunteer there, or have a relative living there. Putting relationships and individuals before tasks has brought measurable value to everyone's life there, and the home has gone from strength to strength, both in terms of the care it offers the people who live there, and its business success, because so many families want its level of care and understanding for their relatives.

The culture at Bruce Lodge didn't change because we all sat down and said we have to do things differently. It is the result of a year's close monitoring of successes and failures, of introducing a way to listen to what matters to people and recording this on one-page profiles, and thinking together how people wanted to use their individual time. The success of our project came down to individuals taking the time to value each other, and to a powerful but flexible framework built from person-centred practices.

Since our work at Bruce Lodge, we have begun to work with a Clinical Commissioning Group and also a national provider to introduce person-centred practices and ISFs. We've continued to learn – learning was a key part of the process at Bruce Lodge – and to see results for both individuals and organisations. We very much hope that people with dementia in all kinds of settings will be able to benefit from person-centred practices and ISFs, so that people can have as much choice and control in their life as possible, and be known and supported as individuals.

APPENDIX

**Personalisation in Care Homes – developing Individual Service Funds
Leadership Team Agenda 26th April
10.00 – 4.00**

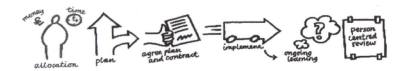

The purpose of the meeting is to:

- Develop a shared understanding of what we want to achieve – what does success look like?
- Review where we are starting from, and progress to date
- Start our communication strategy

Time	What	Who	Outcome	Please come prepared by
10.00	Welcome, introductions, agenda and ground rules	Helen	We know who is in the room, what we are doing today and how we are going to work together	
10.20	Review of the process steps – what are we trying to do?	Helen	We are confident in what the six-stage process means	Having a look at the Dimensions book again!
10.45	Where are we now? Feedback from the baseline evaluations	Gill	We know where we are building from	

cont.

cont.

Time	What	Who	Outcome	Please come prepared by
11.30	Break			
11.45	One-page profiles – meet the team!	Gill and managers	We see the first one-page profiles and the standards/ top tips for one-page profiles in Borough Care	
12.15	What are we planning to do? The project plan so far	Gill and Lisa	We know what the next steps are	
12.30	Lunch			
1.00	What does success look like?	Helen	We develop shared success statements	Think about what you hope to see achieved through this work
2.00	How can we share what we are trying and learning with others? Developing our communication strategy	Helen and Joan	We begin our communication strategy	Think about how you get information at the moment – what channels can we use to communicate this work?
2.45	Break			
3.00	What we need to do before our next meeting on 31st May	Helen	We have a detailed action plan	
3.45	Confirming actions and closing round	Helen	We know what we are each doing next	
4.00	Close			

Figure A1 Example agenda

Borough Care

Tips for developing your one-page profile

Insert your photo to make your one-page profile more personal.

This is particularly helpful if you are sharing your profile with people before you meet them.

Enter your name on top of the profile.

What people like and admire about me...

This needs to be a proud list of your positive qualities, strengths and talents.

Make it clear and avoid using words such as 'usually' or 'sometimes' – be positive.

It is helpful to ask staff, colleagues, friends and family what they like and admire about you.

Do as an exercise in a team meeting, or use positive feedback you have.

What's important to me...

This section needs to have enough detail that someone who does not know you could understand what matters to you, and if you took the names off the profile you could still be identified.

Add things about your whole life that are important to you (your hobbies, interests, passions), as well as things that relate to what's important at work.

Add detail that will help give people an idea of who you are and what you value most, ensuring a good match can be made.

Instead of this

Being organised

Write this

I must get everything I will need for work the following morning organised the evening before, put everything I will need in my briefcase for the next day's meetings and sort out the clothes I will wear. Prepare my to do list for the following day – I love to tick things off as they get done!

How best to support me...

This section includes information on...

What is helpful? What is not?

What others can do to make work time more productive and positive?

Specific areas of development you want to identify for support. For example, you may be working on better time management and have specific things that others can do to support you.

The help you need to create the best environment and outcomes for the people you support.

Instead of this

Stay positive

Write this

I am a glass half full person and it helps me enormously when people look for solutions and not problems. I find it very draining if I am the only optimist.

Figure A2 One-page profile standards for Borough Care

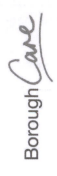

My Home, My Time, My Choice
Personalising Care Homes
One-Page Strategy

Borough *Care*

STOCKPORT
METROPOLITAN BOROUGH COUNCIL

What success means from different perspectives

People living at Bruce Lodge

I am involved in the day-to-day life of where I live in a way that makes sense to me

I am supported by people who know me, and act on what matters to me now, for my future and how I want to be supported

I am listened to and heard, and supported to make choices and decisions

I have individual time each month and choose what I do and who supports me

Staff at Bruce Lodge

Our hobbies and interests are matched to how people living at Bruce Lodge want to spend their individual time

We are listened to and able to contribute to the lives of the people we support, the home and success of the organisation

We get satisfaction from doing a great job and supporting people in a person-centred way on a day-to-day basis, and with their individual hours

Borough Care

We are delivering a person-centred service that people have confidence in, and want to buy

We demonstrate and share good practice in delivering personalised services for people living with dementia in care homes

We know and act on what's working and what's not working for people using and working in our services

Stockport Council

We are commissioning personalised services which are safe and offer real choice for the people living with dementia in Stockport

We are working in active partnership with providers to deliver personalised services for people living in care homes

We share what we are learning locally, regionally and nationally

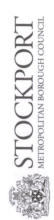

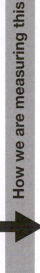
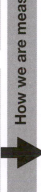

How we are delivering this

The Leadership Team Borough Care and Stockport Council with HSA

Project team one-page profiles
Working/Not working
Doughnut – to clarify responsibilities in delivering this
Communication chart – sharing learning locally, regionally and nationally

Staff one-page profiles
Matching staff
Working/Not working

One-page profiles
Communication charts and decision-making agreements
Working/Not working
Outcomes for individual time
Learning logs (for individual time)
Matching staff

How we are measuring this

Increase in the scores from Dementia Mapping and Observation Schedule
Increase in scores from Progress for Providers
Percentage of actions achieved from Dementia Mapping recommendations
Number of places/ways where information about this has been shared
a) Internally
b) externally (regionally and nationally)

Percentage of people living at Bruce Lodge whose individual time is delivered by key worker. We are looking for staff to be chosen individually and not expecting this to always be the keyworker
Analysis of how the 2 hours are used per person. We are expecting to see variety, for example some people having their 2 hours a month in 4 half-hour sessions
Percentage of people who use their individual time outside of Bruce Lodge. We are looking for a high percentage of people to use their time to be in the community
Range of creative options (versus traditional options) tried to enable people to use their 2 hours in the way that they want

Number of staff with one-page profiles that meet standards
Matching staff used for each individual based on how they want to spend their individual 2 hours
Percentage of Learning Logs used to capture learning from how people spent their individual time
Increase in scores from Progress for Providers

Number of people with one-page profiles that meet standards, with Working/Not working
Number of people with communication charts/decision-making agreements
Number of people who have clear specified outcome for using their 2 hours individual time
Increase in scores from Dementia Care Map

Figure A3 One Page Strategy

My Home, My Time, My Choice: Personalising Care Homes Pilot Project

Dashboard

	April	May	June	July	August	Sept	Oct	Nov	Dec	Jan
How we are measuring this for people living at Bruce Lodge										
Number of people with one-page profiles and working/not working										
Communication charts/decision-making agreements										
How we are measuring this for staff at Bruce Lodge										
Staff one-page profiles (total)										
Staff "if I could, I would" (total)										
Number of completed learning logs (in month)										
How we are measuring this for the leadership team										
Number of individual sessions done by keyworker (in month)										
Number of people using their 2 hours outside Bruce Lodge (total that month)										
Number of completed comments cards (in month)										
Number of responses to comments cards (in month)										
Blogs written/videos										
Hits on Blog (Stockport)										
Written stories										
Borough Care hits on web page										
HSA Blog										
Tweets										
Facebook										

Figure A4 Dashboard

Dementia Care Mapping (DCM): 23 behaviour category codes

A: articulation–communicating using verbal or nonverbal techniques

B: borderline–being awake and engaged but as a passive observer

C: cool–disengaged from environment

D: doing for self–all self-care actions

E: self-expression–using music/art/objects to express

F: food–anything relating to food and fluids

G: going back–reminiscence

I: intellectual–use of intellectual skills

J: joints–exercise, not walking

K: kum and go–walking

L: leisure, such as watching television or reading

N: land of nod–asleep

O: objects–holding and/or interacting with objects

P: physical–personal or physical care

R: religion–forms of religious expression

S: sexual expression–including cuddling

T: timulation–engaging through senses

U: unresponded to–not receiving response to communication

V: vocation–work-like activity

W: withstanding–contact with self, self-stimulation

X: x-cretion–everything about excretion

Y: yourself–interacting in the absence of others

Z: zero option–fits no other option

INDEX